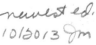

Date Due

Suicide and Depression in Late Life

An Einstein Psychiatry Publication

Publication Series of the Department of Psychiatry
Albert Einstein College of Medicine of Yeshiva University
New York, NY

Suicide and Depression in Late Life

Critical Issues in Treatment, Research, and Public Policy

Edited by

GARY J. KENNEDY

John Wiley & Sons, Inc.

New York • Chichester • Brisbane • Toronto • Singapore

This text is printed on acid-free paper.

This publication is designed to provide accurate and authoritative
information in regard to the subject matter covered. It is sold
with the understanding that the publisher is not engaged in
rendering professional services. If legal, accounting, medical,
psychological, or any other expert assistance is required, the
services of a competent professional person should be sought.

Library of Congress Cataloging-in-Publication Data:

Suicide and depression in late life : critical issues in treatment,
    research, and public policy / edited by Gary J. Kennedy.
          p.   cm. — (Publication series of the Department of Psychiatry
    Albert Einstein College of Medicine of Yeshiva University ; 13)
       Includes index.
       ISBN 0-471-12913-5 (alk. paper)
       1. Depression in old age.   2. Aged—Suicidal behavior.
    I. Kennedy, Gary J., 1948–   . II. Series: Einstein psychiatry
    publication ; 13.
    RC537.5.S85   1996
    618.97′68527—dc20   95-37313

Printed in the United States of America

10   9   8   7   6   5   4   3   2   1

Contributors

F. M. Baker, M.D., MPH Erasmus University Medical School, Rotterdam, The Netherlands.

Alexander J. Botsis, M.D. Senior Lecturer, Department of Psychiatry, Athens School of Medicine, Athens General Army Hospital, Athens, Greece.

Rama P. Coomaraswamy, M.D. Assistant Professor, Department of Psychiatry, Albert Einstein College of Medicine, Montefiore Medical Center, Bronx, New York.

Donald P. Hay, M.D. Associate Professor of Psychiatry and Director, Geriatric Psychiatry Inpatient Program, St. Louis University School of Medicine, Department of Psychiatry and Human Behavior and Medical Center, St. Louis, Missouri.

Linda K. Hay, Ph.D. Assistant Professor and Director of Psychological Services in Division of Geriatric Psychiatry, St. Louis University School of Medicine, Department of Psychiatry and Human Behavior and Medical Center, St. Louis, Missouri.

Gary J. Kennedy, M.D. Associate Professor, Department of Psychiatry, and Director, Division of Geriatric Psychiatry, Albert Einstein College of Medicine, Montefiore Medical Center, Bronx, New York.

Robert Lowinger, M.D. Assistant Professor and Assistant Director, Division of Geriatric Psychiatry, Albert Einstein College of Medicine, Montefiore Medical Center, Bronx, New York.

Helen Metz, Ph.D. Assistant Professor, Department of Psychiatry, Albert Einstein College of Medicine, Montefiore Medical Center, Bronx, New York.

Robert Plutchik, Ph.D. Professor Emeritus, Department of Psychiatry, Albert Einstein College of Medicine, Montefiore Medical Center, Bronx, New York.

Joseph Richman, Ph.D. Professor Emeritus, Department of Psychiatry, Albert Einstein College of Medicine, Montefiore Medical Center, Bronx, New York.

Lon S. Schneider, M.D. Associate Professor of Psychiatry and Neurology, University of Southern California School of Medicine, Los Angeles, California.

Herman M. van Praag, M.D., Ph.D. Professor and Chairman, Academic Psychiatric Center, University of Limburg, Maastricht, The Netherlands.

Marcella Bakur Weiner, Ed.D. Professor (Adjunct), Department of Psychology, Brooklyn College of the City University of New York, Brooklyn, New York.

A Note on the Series

Psychiatry is in a state of flux. The excitement springs in part from internal changes, such as the development and official acceptance (at least in the United States) of an operationalized, multi-axial classification system of behavioral disorders (the DSM-IV), the increasing sophistication of methods to measure abnormal human behavior, and the impressive expansion of biological and psychological treatment modalities. Exciting developments are also taking place in fields relating to psychiatry; in molecular (brain) biology, genetics, brain imaging, drug development, epidemiology, experimental psychology, to mention only a few striking examples.

More generally speaking, psychiatry is moving, still relatively slowly, but irresistibly from a more philosophical, contemplative orientation to that of an empirical science. From the 1950s on, biological psychiatry has been a major catalyst of that process. It provided the mother discipline with a third cornerstone, that is, neurobiology, the other two being psychology and medical sociology. In addition, it forced the profession into the direction of standardization of diagnoses and of assessment of abnormal behavior. Biological psychiatry provided not only with a new basic science and with new treatment modalities, but also with the tools, the methodology, and the mentality to operate within the confines of an empirical science, the only framework in which a medical discipline can survive.

In other fields of psychiatry, too, one discerns a gradual trend toward scientification. Psychological treatment techniques are standardized and manuals developed to make these skills more easily transferable. Methods registering treatment outcome—traditionally used in the behavioral/cognitive field—are now more and more requested and, hence, developed for dynamic forms of psychotherapy as well. Social and community psychiatry, until the 1960s were more firmly rooted in humanitarian ideals and social awareness than in empirical studies, profited greatly from its liaison with the social sciences and the expansion of psychiatric epidemiology.

Let there be no misunderstanding: Empiricism does *not imply* that it is only the measurable that counts. Psychiatry would be mutilated if it would neglect that which cannot be captured by numbers. It *does imply* that what is measurable should be measured. progress in psychiatry is dependent on ideas and on experiment. Their linkage is inseparable.

This Series, published under the auspices of the Department of Psychiatry of the Albert Einstein College of Medicine, Montefiore Medical Center, is meant to keep track of important developments in our profession, to summarize what has been achieved in particular fields, and to bring together the viewpoints obtained from disparate vantage points—in short, to capture some of the ongoing excitement in modern psychiatry, both in its clinical and experimental dimensions. The Department of Psychiatry at Albert Einstein College of Medicine hosts the Series, but naturally welcomes contributions from others.

Bernie Mazel originally generated the idea for the series—an ambitious plan which we all felt was worthy of pursuit. The edifice of psychiatry is impressive, but still somewhat flawed in its foundations. May this Series contribute to consolidation of its infrastructure.

—HERMAN M. VAN PRAAG, M.D., PHD.
Professor and Chairman
Academic Psychiatric Center
University of Limburg
Maastricht
The Netherlands

Foreword

The last act of life is not always its merriest. Responsibilities may be diminished, expectations may be few. The children are away, sometimes far away; friends expire; many lose their partner. The body has become less reliable, and physical appearance may have become less appealing. The credit balance of one's life accomplishments may, in retrospect, seem small. Feelings of self-deprecation may flourish under such conditions and feelings of emptiness and boredom may arise, with life reduced to little more than waiting for death to come.

The understanding and support available to the older person in these circumstances may be less than hoped for. "Don't keep harping on your troubles!" is the message frequently communicated. Few friends or family members enjoy discussions of death and dying. Mentioning a host of physical complaints makes one appear to be a hypochondriac. Feelings of loneliness may blossom when the attempts by older people to discuss their very real concerns are rejected.

Feelings of emptiness, boredom, and loneliness do not promote good mental health. In addition, the actual neuronal functioning of the brain declines with age, leading to defects in mood regulation. As a result, there is an increased risk of depression if the stress level of the older person rises.

I realize that this is a gloomy picture of old age. The aging process does not necessarily proceed that way, but the older patient experiences some or all of these losses frequently enough to predict a high risk of depression in the elderly. And indeed, this is the reality.

Is depression generally recognized as such? The answer is no. In medical practice, many depressions remain undiagnosed and untreated. The chance of that happening increases with age. Comorbidity with other syndromes may disguise the depression. In other cases, the saddened mood is thought to be understandable, and hence the possibility of a treatable depression is ignored. Interestingly, this line of reasoning is not followed in other kinds of illnesses. For example, if a patient who smokes, eats too much, and exercises too little has hypertension, the fact that the physician understands the genesis of the disorder is not considered a hindrance to therapy. Apparently, psychiatry still occupies an exceptional position in medicine.

Is depression in the elderly, if recognized, treated adequately? Often it is not. Dosage of antidepressants may be too low and duration of treatment too short, due to fear of side effects or incompatibility with other medications. Psychotherapy is offered too infrequently. Psychodynamic psychotherapy is sometimes considered contraindicated or useless in the elderly, although the reasoning behind this thinking has never convinced me.

Experience is still limited as to the usefulness of cognitive therapy and interpersonal psychotherapy in this population; meanwhile underfunding and a shortage of mental health specialists remain obstacles to adequate access to therapy.

Are systematic attempts being made to enrich the experiences of those elderly living alone, in nursing homes, or in homes for the aged, to make such lives more rewarding, more colorful, more stimulating? Again, efforts are inadequate. Funding is insufficient and volunteer organizations have lost their appeal as women—the primary constituents of traditional volunteer pools—have sought "real" (paid) work.

The tone of this Foreword is in a minor key. I believe my appraisal is no exaggeration. The number of elderly people is rapidly increasing; their life span is lengthening; and with added years of life, illness is a more frequent companion. Because physicians are not trained sufficiently to address these problems and must care for patients in a setting of inadequate social support, the elderly may be at increased risk of depression and further mental and physical deterioration.

Funds, the medical profession cannot provide; knowledge, it can and should provide. Hence, the book you are about to read will be extremely useful. The subject matter as well as the quality of this book makes its reading well worth the effort. It provides a comprehensive review of depression in the elderly. Old age is accompanied by many infirmities and losses that cannot be avoided, but depression is treatable and both its diagnosis and treatment are expertly discussed in this volume.

Being well on my way to seniority myself, I am pleased that this book has been written, and I hope that it will contribute to a better life for many of my fellow senior citizens.

HERMAN M. VAN PRAAG, M.D., PH.D.
Academic Psychiatric Center
University of Limburg
Maastricht
The Netherlands

Preface

Despite major advances in the health and economic well-being of older Americans, in the 1980s late-life suicide became more prevalent than at any time in the previous 50 years. Modern medicine's extension of life beyond meaning is frequently cited as the cause of this troubling phenomenon and has resulted in decisions to forgo lifesaving treatment and the establishment of living wills. However, there is little scientific evidence that loss of life's meaning or social stature accounts for even a significant minority of elderly suicides.

Large-scale epidemiological surveys of suicide and depression have added little to our understanding of the causes of suicidal behavior in late life or how we might help the vulnerable individual. As a result, there are no accepted estimates of the number of aged community residents whose suicidal ideas might be ameliorated with appropriate medical attention. This is particularly regrettable in light of the growth in diagnostic procedures and safe, effective treatments for both mild and severe depression among the elderly.

The notion that suicide and depression are often reasonable responses to loss and disability in old age, rather than a manifestation of treatable mental illness does not represent informed social policy. It reinforces the older adult's wish to avoid being labeled as mentally ill. Already, older adults seek mental health care far below the most conservative estimates of mental illness in late life. A preoccupation with the loss of autonomy coupled with an avoidance of the stigma of mental illness makes present mental health services ill equipped to meet the rising morbidity and mortality associated with late-life suicidal behavior.

The authors explore the biology, psychology, epidemiology, and sociology of depression and suicidal behavior in late life as well as ethical principles that underlie clinical research and therapeutic intervention. The range of treatment including environmental manipulation, psychotherapy, family counseling, medications, and electroconvulsive therapy is reviewed, and guidelines for effective interventions are provided. The limits of existing scientific data and social policy are detailed. Readers will gain a better understanding of the dilemma presented by the older adult's thoughts of death in relation both to mental illness and rational expectations for the end of the life span.

GARY J. KENNEDY, M.D.
Director, Division of Geriatric Psychiatry
Albert Einstein College of Medicine,
Montefiore Medical Center
Bronx, New York

Contents

PART I
Critical Issues in Clinical Science

1

Epidemiology and Inferences Regarding the Etiology of Late-Life Suicide

GARY J. KENNEDY,
HELEN METZ, AND
ROBERT LOWINGER

More than 20 years after Brown and Sherman (1972) called for a wholly new conception of self-inflicted death, the literature on late-life suicide continues to advance slowly because of methodological and theoretical difficulties. Although the highest rates of suicide are found in the elderly, adolescent suicide and adult homicide have received considerably greater attention (Woodbury, Manton, & Blazer, 1988). The increasing rate of late-life suicides as well as the growing number of older adults in the United States makes this lack of information particularly troubling. Sociologists and journalists assert that the increase reflects advanced medical procedures, which have changed the dream of long life into the nightmare of prolonged death. In contrast, clinical scientists argue that depressive disorders are the driving force behind late-life suicide. Chronic illness and alcoholism have also been cited as well as a greater social acceptance of suicide among the elderly (Sorenson, 1991). Studies of late-life psychopathology offer little to expand our understanding of suicide among older adults, those 65 and older (Holden, 1992; Lindsey, 1991).

As a consequence, inferences to explain the increase in late-life suicides as well as the raw data on which rates are based are both problematic. Table 1–1 displays the commonly accepted risk profile (both
social and psychopathological components) of suicidality among older
Americans.

RATES AND TRENDS

Suicides among older adults declined by 42% between 1950 and 1980
(McCall, 1991). But by 1987, the rate of 21.6 suicides per 100,000 older
adults exceeded that observed immediately prior to the institution of
Medicare in 1965, reversing the downward trend in elderly suicide
which had started in 1933 (Tolchin, 1989). Between 1981 and 1987, the
rate of late-life suicides increased by 25% despite substantial advances
in the economic and health status of older adults (Osgood, 1989). In
1986, suicide was the 10th leading cause of death among adults aged 65
and older (Blazer, Bachar, & Manton, 1986) and ranked after falls and
automobile accidents as the third most common cause of death from injury. By 1988, there were more than 6,000 late-life suicides per year
(National Center for Health Statistics, 1990), a rate that left the decade
of the 1980s with 60,000 older adult suicides (Meehan, Saltzberg, &
Sattin, 1991).

Although older persons make up 12% of the population, they account
for one third of all suicides (Dyer, 1992). And there is little doubt that
present rates, based on death certificates, are an underestimate (Miller,
1978). For every completed late-life suicide, there are no less than four

TABLE 1–1
Characteristics of Older Adults at Increased Risk for Suicide

Sociodemographic	Clinical	Historical
White, male	Depression	Previous attempt
Divorced, widowed	Alcoholism	Family history
Lives alone	Chronic pain	Lethality of attempt
Recent life change event	Poor health	Rescued by accident
Anniversary of loss	Disability	Firearms possession
75 or older		Expressed intent

Note: Adapted from "Psychogeriatric Emergencies," by G. J. Kennedy and R. Lowinger,
1993, in L. Pousada (Ed.), *Clinics in Geriatric Medicine, 9,* 641–654. Copyright 1993 by
W. B. Saunders and Co. Adapted by permission.

attempts (Parkin & Stengal, 1965). There is no reliable estimate of the number of chronically ill, isolated elderly adults who attempt or complete passive suicide through self-neglect (Osgood, 1992). Gallup estimates that as many as 600,000 adults aged 60 or older have considered suicide in the previous 6 months (Gallup, 1992). Even if the percentage of elderly suicides does not grow, the absolute number of late-life suicides will double over the next 40 years (Whanger, 1989).

GENDER

In 1988, suicide rates between ages 80 and 84 ran from a low of 1.2/100,000 among African American women to a high of 72.6/100,000 among white males. Male gender is a powerful risk factor across the life span. For all ages combined, the ratio of male to female suicides is 4 to 1, but in the 85-and-older group the ratio is 12 to 1 (National Center for Health Statistics, 1990). Above age 65, 80% of suicides are male (Dyer, 1992). Gender through an interaction with age and depression also affects suicide attempts. Men seem more likely to attempt suicide following a later-onset depressive disorder, whereas women are more likely to attempt suicide with early onset of depression (Bron, Strack, & Rudolph, 1991). White males have been preponderant among elderly suicides since the beginning of the 20th century (McIntosh, 1985), but suicide rates in African American men also increased between 1968 and 1981. Table 1–2 shows the change in suicide rate among older adults from the low point in 1981 to the most recently available 1988 data from the National Center for Health Statistics. The comparison between 1981 and 1988 indicates a substantial increase in late-life suicides, not only among black men but also among black and white women and white men (National Center for Health Statistics, 1990). Figures showing a decrease may well be spurious because the number of deaths is so small.

SOCIOECONOMIC INFERENCES

Another explanation for the high rates of elderly suicide particularly in older white males relative to other groups has to do with role and status loss related to retirement (Maris, 1969; McIntosh & Santos, 1981) and lack of companionship. In 1986, the rate for divorced men was 3.2 times that for married men and 18.9 times that for married women (Meehan, Saltzberg, & Sattin, 1991). This seems to confirm Durkheim's

TABLE 1–2
Suicides per 100,000 Older Americans by Race and Gender

All Older Adults Age	65–69	70–74	75–79	80–84	85 +
1981	15.6	16.9	18.3	19.0	17.7
1988	17.2	20.0	24.5	28.0	20.5
% Change	10.2	18.3	33.8	47.3	15.8
White Men					
1981	27.2	33.8	41.2	48.6	53.6
1988	32.0	39.8	55.3	72.6	65.8
% Change	17.6	17.7	34.2	49.3	22.7
Black Men					
1981	10.5	8.6	18.2	17.5	12.7
1988	13.3	12.3	18.6	15.7	10.0
% Change	26.6	43.0	2.1	−10.2[a]	−21.2[b]
White Women					
1981	7.8	6.6	6.7	5.0	3.7
1988	7.0	7.5	7.6	7.1	5.3
% Change	10.2	13.6	13.4	42.0	43.2
Black Women					
1981	2.1	4.3	1.6	NA	1.8
1988	2.6	1.3	1.4	1.2	NA
% Change	23.8	−69.7[c]	−12.5[d]	—	—

[a] Compared with the 1987 rate of 25.0, the increase is 42.8%.

[b] Compared with the 1987 rate of 13.0, the increase is 2.3%.

[c] Based on the 1980 rate of 1.5 and the 1987 rate of 2.9, the increase is 48.2%; based on the 1982 rate of 1.9 and the 1987 rate of 2.9, the increase is 34.4%.

[d] Compared with the 1987 rate of 2.5, the increase is 56.2%.

Source: National Center for Health Statistics. (1991). Vital statistics of the United States, 1988: Vol. II. *Mortality, Part A.* Washington, DC: Public Health Service.

observation, reported in 1890, that in regard to suicide men benefited more from marriage than women (Durkheim, 1891/1951). Loss of spouse, excessive use of alcohol, depression, experience with suicide of a friend or relative and no fear of retribution may be significant in accounting for high rates among white males. But systematic surveys that attempted to tease apart the contributions of age, gender, and race are far from adequate in explaining the reasons for elevated rates among white males (Murphy, Wetzel, Robins, & McEvoy, 1992).

The literature on retirement, career development, and life satisfaction offers opposing views (Atchley, 1980). The conditions surrounding retirement rather than the event itself are often more important in determining the psychological impact of giving up work. For example, differences in life satisfaction following retirement are based on whether leaving the workplace was mandatory or voluntary; the occupational level of the position surrendered; opportunities for future employment, volunteer work, or leisure pursuits; and financial status. In addition, the assumption that shedding social roles and ties has a negative impact on older adults may be incorrect. Disengagement (Cummings & Henry, 1961) theory asserts that giving up social roles and responsibilities for a more self-centered focus may result in greater life satisfaction.

Social isolation is an accepted risk factor for suicide. Barraclough (1971) found living alone to be the most highly correlated social variable in late-life suicide. Loneliness was one of the earliest reasons identified behind late-life suicide attempts (Batchelor & Napier, 1953). However, the existing studies of late-life suicidality fail to distinguish between real and perceived social isolation. And, among older adults who live alone, few consider themselves isolated and fewer still attempt suicide. Data on the perceived adequacy of social support is available in the depression literature but not that dealing with suicide.

PERIOD AND COHORT EFFECTS

Characteristics of the epoch (period) and generation (cohort) under observation influence the prevalence and etiology of clinical phenomena. For example, the relatively low prevalence of depression among older compared with younger age groups in the 1980s is thought to be the result of a cohort phenomenon rather than some aspect of the period of observation (Klerman et al. (1985). The present cohort of young adults also shows a higher rate of suicide than their grandparents at the younger ages (Haas & Hendin, 1983). Based on analyses of period, cohort, age, gender, and race effects on suicide rates between 1962 and 1982, Woodbury et al. (1988) suggested that rates among elderly white males would stabilize, not increasing until the cohorts born after 1947 reached 65. They found little evidence to suggest that physical disability due to chronic illness and mental disorders, which are higher among older women than men, could account for the relatively stable rate of suicides among women. Thus both the low rates for women and the high rates for men over the 20-year period beginning in 1962 were more consistent with social than with psychobiological etiology. They further speculated that age predominated in white male rates but that cohort effects predominated in nonwhite males. Thus white male rates should remain stable, whereas nonwhite rates should decline. However, it remains to be seen if older adult cohorts passing into their 7th and 8th decades in the 1990s will experience the same flattening of the suicide rate curve observed in previous cohorts.

Using post-World War II annual time series analysis, McCall (1991) generated data suggesting that relative societal affluence was associated with suicide trends among elderly white males. Easterlin (1986) hypothesized that a large birth cohort, particularly in relation to the rest of the population, has economic and employment consequences: The larger the cohort, the more difficulty it will find competing for resources and jobs. Unfortunately, neither period nor cohort effects in this instance are much of a guide to etiology given the increase in suicides at a time of advanced social and economic well-being for older Americans. Moreover, the increasing prevalence of depression and suicide at younger ages, coupled with the increasing number of older adults in the U.S. population, may lead to a substantial increase in late-life suicide into the 21st century. Thus the psychopathology of younger adults and the coming socioeconomic-demographic shifts in the next century suggest that both period and cohort effects will make suicide prevention an imperative public health concern.

METHODS OF SUICIDE

Among both men and women, firearms are the most common method of suicidal death. Suicide by firearms is also more common in the elderly than among persons less than 65. The presence of a firearm in the home increases the risk of suicide more than fourfold even after controlling for variables such as living along or the use of psychotropic medications or alcohol (Kellerman et al., 1992). Suicides by firearms increased by 10% between 1980 and 1986 among older men and women combined. In 1992, more than 65% of suicides among older persons were firearm related (Osgood, 1992).

After reviewing suicide rates in the five boroughs of New York City, Marzuk et al. (1992) concluded that the differences between the boroughs were almost wholly explained by differences in the accessibility to lethal methods. Suicide rates from firearms had fallen since the institution of strict handgun control measures across the boroughs. Common household methods of death including hanging, suffocation, knifing, and poisoning with nonprescription medications varied little from borough to borough. Falling from heights, overdose of prescription medications, and carbon monoxide poisoning were the principal reasons for the differences.

Among residents of nursing homes, self-starvation may be the most common method of suicide. However, the self-starving persons denied that their behavior was suicidal, saying "they were just helping God along" (Osgood, 1992).

Hawton and Fagg (1990) studied patients referred to a general hospital following deliberate self-poisoning or self-injury. Close to 25% of the attempters (more men than women) had consumed alcohol within 6 hours of the event and more than 25% had made previous attempts. Interestingly enough, the rates of self-poisoning remained stable despite a significant decline in the use of barbiturates during the period of study. The decrease in barbiturates was made up for with the use of nonopiate analgesics and other prescription drugs, also reported by Lindsey (1986). The number of attempts in the 55- to 64-year age group was almost double that of the group that was 65 and older. However, although the attempt rate was greater among the younger patients, the fatality rate was greater among the older. Whereas the risk of suicide attempts declined with age, the risk of fatality increased (Hawton & Fagg, 1990). Thus advancing age may offer less likelihood that survival following a suicide attempt would have a cathartic effect observed by van Praag and Plutchik (1985) among younger adults.

In England and the Netherlands, the detoxification (reduction of carbon monoxide) of coal gas was followed by a reduction in suicides. However, there appeared to be a compensatory rise in medication overdoses suggesting a substitution of methods in response to a change in availability of legal means. Reducing the accessibility of suicidal methods may genuinely reduce the suicidal attempts among impulsive or ambivalent individuals but does not appear to change the risk for those determined to kill themselves. However, risk factors such as access to firearms and prescription drugs are alterable (Marzuk et al., 1992). Even if restricting access to more legal methods results in substitution of less lethal methods, the net effect on mortality would be beneficial.

GEOGRAPHIC PATTERNS

To compare nations with varying prevalence of suicide, Pritchard (1992) developed a "ratio of ratios" in which the ratio of all-age suicides to the elderly ratio was compared by year to obtain a measure of change. Since 1974, suicide rates among American men increased among all age groups, but the greatest increases were among the aged. Overall suicide rates fell among younger women, but not among the elderly. The United States ranked eighth in prevalence of suicide among elderly men but fourth in the relative increase compared with all-age suicides. Only Norway, Finland, and Austria experienced a greater change in the ratio of ratios. Although late-life suicides increased across the developed nations of Western Europe and the United Kingdom, the rates among older American men and women were among the worst.

Between 1980 and 1986, the rate of late-life suicides decreased in the northeast United States but rose by more than 20% across the southern, western, and north-central areas. In 1986, there were 13.6 suicides among 100,000 older adults in the Northeast compared to a high of 23.7 in the South (Marzuk et al., 1992).

PHYSICAL ILLNESS

Physical illness has a central role in late-life suicide. Among individuals 60 years of age and older, as many as 70% may have had a physical illness directly contributing to the completion of suicide (Mackensie & Popkin, 1987). And as many as 50% of attempters also have substantial health problems (Owens, 1990). Chronic heart and lung conditions as well as diseases of the central nervous system are the most frequently cited examples (Horton-Deutsch, Clark, & Farran, 1992). In a retrospective study of late-life suicides in Chicago, Clark (1992) found that 20% of the sample had seen their physician within 24 hours of death. Interviews with the physicians revealed that their patients had presented vague physical symptoms, and when inquiries about mental symptoms were attempted, the patients demurred. In contrast, their families recalled difficulties with depression and alcohol as well as prescription drugs. However, there are no available studies comparing the prevalence of completed suicide, attempts, or ideas among older adults with physical illness and disability. Neither do we have any data on why some physically ill older adults attempt suicide whereas others do not.

Conwell, Caine, and Olsen (1990) and Murphy (1977) offer data to suggest that some fraction of late-life suicides are the result of the individual's perception of a terminal illness that cannot be verified either by acquittances or physicians. However, it is unclear whether these distorted perceptions are simply delusional. Finally, no studies have addressed the questions of recency of onset or extent of associated disability, which have clear effects on depressive symptoms and may also impel suicidal ideas. It may be that it is not the perception of illness that is distorted in these individuals but rather the extent to which they view their condition as hopeless. Hopelessness is a significant predictor of suicidal ideas among depressed older outpatients (Hill, Gallager, Thompson, & Ishida, 1988) and subsequent completed suicide in younger inpatients (Beck, Steer, Kovacs, & Garrison, 1985); and it is more frequent among older than younger community residents (Green, 1981).

EXCESSES OF MODERN MEDICINE

Angell (1990) and others (Kevorkian cure, 1990) suggest that medical advances have extended life beyond meaning so that older suicides "fear living more than dying because they dread becoming prisoners of technology" (p. A17). Loebel et al. have also reported a significant relationship between suicide and anticipation of confinement to a nursing home (Loebel, Loebel, Dager, Centerwall, & Reay, 1991). The "Kevorkian cure" of physician-assisted suicide is perhaps the most troubling example of anticipatory suicide. Quill's (1991) report of assisted suicide, "Death and Dignity," describes a lengthy, deeply informed patient-physician relationship that represents the opposite end of the spectrum from Kevorkian's cases where neither the patient's suffering nor the physician's knowledge of his patient's condition seems compelling.

Miller (1978) identified the threshold of suicide as a "level of unbearability" that is a subjective response reflecting the accumulation of life experiences, resources, and coping mechanisms. However, the distinction between a rational preference for death over unbearable disability, and a suicidal impulse due to mental illness in late life is not easily determined. Terms such as "subintentioned death" (Shneidman, 1963), "hidden suicide" (Merloo, 1968), and "indirect life-threatening behavior" (Nelson & Farberow, 1977) appear to describe masked or passive suicide, but the range of behaviors that might be considered indirectly threatening has yet to be satisfactorily delimited for research purposes. Conwell, Caine, and

Olsen (1990), who reported that six of a series of eight elderly suicides had delusional concerns over cancer and had approached their physician about these concerns, further questions the validity of rational suicide. Despite the popularity of *Final Exit* (Humphrey, 1991), a how-to book for prospective suicides, there is little evidence that physically ill elderly adults suicide in the absence of a depressive or other mental disorder (Shaffer, 1993).

These problematic inferences are also evident in the area of adolescent suicide. In 1982, "anti-mental illness" model prevailed with various constituency groups committed to the notion that suicide resulted from social forces rather than from "medical problems." A significant minority of suicides are thought to occur in the presence of others, and the survivors' guilt over missing the warning signs contributes to biasing reports toward calling them accidents rather than suicides. Susan J. Blumenthal, as cited by Bakken, states, "I think this phenomenon is linked to the stigma that still surrounds mental illness in our society (Bakken, 1991). Families would rather believe that there are external forces operating, like the influence of the media, rather than that their child is suffering from mental illness and that they did not receive treatment for the disorder" (pp. 28–32).

MEDIA PRESENTATION

Etzersdorfer, Sonnek, and Nagel-Kuess's (1992) survey of subway suicides in Vienna suggested a genuine connection between the prominence of press coverage and both the overall rates and choice of lethal methods. The Austrian Association for Suicide Prevention promulgated guidelines for the press that resulted in reductions of space given to the reports and in the frequency with which suicide appeared on the front page. A reduction in front-page reportage was associated with a reduction both in total suicides by year and in subway suicides.

Rosenberg, Eddy, Wolpert, and Broumas (1989) discuss the portrayal of adolescent suicide in the media and among the victim's peers. They emphasize the importance of not dramatizing the event so as not to foster imitative suicidal attempts. Labeling suicidal thought as normative may increase rather than decrease the prevalence of suicidal ideas. Instead, the distress that leads to suicide should be acknowledged and portrayed as a missed opportunity to get help. This avoids painting the individual as a hero who gained control in desperate circumstances or as a victim with no escape other than death. The mystification of suicide and the stigma that the elderly are useless are among the greatest impediments to dealing with late-life suicide (Barr, 1992).

Companion pieces from the *New England Journal of Medicine* illustrate the importance of these seemingly superficial semantic options. Quill, Cassel, and Meier (1992) use the phrase "physician-assisted suicide" for individuals who are hopelessly and soon to be terminally ill, whereas Brody (1992) in contrast uses "assisted death." Labeling the assisted death of a terminally ill individual as a suicide risks influencing public opinion to be more accepting of genuine suicides of depressed or misguided individuals who are neither hopelessly nor terminally ill.

PUBLIC OPINION ON THE ETIOLOGY
OF LATE-LIFE SUICIDE

In the clinical literature, depression and physical illness are the more common factors in late-life suicide. In contrast, the Gallup Organization (1992) found that the elderly cite loneliness as the major reason why an older person might consider or commit suicide. Financial problems, poor health, depression, excess alcohol, "not taking prescription drugs properly," feelings of worthlessness, and isolate behavior were also cited. When asked where a suicidal friend could go for help, however, only 13% of the sample identified a physician or clergy and nearly 25% could not identify any source of help. Of individuals who reported a suicide attempt, most described themselves as not very religious. More than three quarters had not talked about suicide before the attempt. Only 13% had sought any form of help before attempting suicide.

When asked about select attitudes toward late-life suicide, 42% agreed that physicians should assist in suicide when there is incurable illness or intractable suffering. More than a third agreed that late-life suicide should be viewed differently from teenage suicide. More than a quarter of the sample agreed that late-life suicide was a personal decision in which others should not be involved.

INFERENCES FROM THE
NEUROBIOLOGY OF SUICIDALITY

The decrease in brain serotonergic function, which has been associated with depressive disorders, panic disorder, and suicidal behavior in younger adults, is also thought to be associated with normal aging in part because the activity of monoamine oxidase that metabolizes serotonin increases with age. Coccaro et al. (1989) suggest that serotonin acts as a "brake" against suicidal impulses. This suggests an age-related risk of suicide that may be dissociated from conventional categories of mental disorders. But if serotonin is the brake, alcohol is surely the accelerator (Holden, 1992).

Using data from the St. Louis Epidemiologic Catchment Area (ECA) study, Murphy et al. (1992) described six risk factors associated with suicide among alcoholics. These included, in order of frequency, recent heavy drinking, self-report or hearsay evidence of suicidal talk, lack of social support, major depressive disorder, unemployment, living alone, and presence of a serious medical problem. The frequency of risk factors differed significantly when compared with ECA living alcoholics and nonalcoholic individuals with a major depressive disorder who committed suicide. The authors point out that the risk factors were relatively subacute if not long-standing and at least in the case of major depressive disorder potentially reversible. Moreover, the accumulation of risk factors could be used as a guide to preventive intervention even among alcoholics who refused treatment of the primary disorder.

The mean age of the group under study was 47 years, which raises questions about the utility of the approach to older drinkers. In contrast, Hemenway, Solnick, and Colditz's (1993) study showing a marked relationship between smoking and suicide demonstrated an increased relative risk for women aged 60 and above. The authors suggest that smoking, as a self-medicating behavior to counter depression is an indirect risk factor for suicide.

INFERENCES REGARDING MAJOR MENTAL DISORDERS AND SUICIDE

Data from clinical series indicate that a depressive episode is present in a range from about 67% (Gurland & Cross, 1983) to more than 90% (Conwell, Melanie, & Caine, 1990) of older adults who commit suicide. Severity of depressive symptoms rather than the presence of psychosis correlates positively with completed suicide (Clayton, 1985). And while estimates of the prevalence of depressive disorders in late life vary depending on the definition of a case, there is no question but that the majority of depressive episodes in older adults go untreated (Brown & Sherman, 1972; Hershfeld & Klerman, 1979).

However, information from community samples suggests that depressive disorders may play a less prominent role in late-life suicide. Weissman, Klerman, Markowitz, & Ouellette (1989) reported the frequency of suicidal thoughts and a history of suicide attempts among participants of the ECA studies. Among those not meeting diagnostic criteria for any psychiatric disorder, 15% "thought a lot about death," 4% "felt so low they thought about committing suicide," 3% "felt like they wanted to die," and 1% reported a past suicide attempt. Surprisingly, no relationship between depressive disorder and suicide attempts or suicidal thoughts was observed. Panic attacks and panic disorders, but not advances age, were related to suicidal ideas and attempts. However, the ECA diagnostic algorithm purposefully excluded individuals from the diagnostic rubric with physical illness or a disability that might be etiologic of mental symptoms. This effectively reduces to a minimum those older adults whom clinical studies suggest would have reported suicidal ideas.

Although not all older adults who express suicidal ideas attempt suicide, it is thought that most elderly suicides have verbalized the thought (Osgood, 1985). Thus some measure of suicidal thinking seems the most reasonably proxy measure with which to generate hypotheses about the etiology and prevention of suicidal behavior. Unfortunately, the extant community survey databases do not contain these data. The Established Populations for the Epidemiologic Studies of the Elderly Resource Data Book (Cornoni-Huntley, Brock, Ostfeld, Taylor, & Wallace, 1986) contains extensive information on mood, cognition, functional ability, tobacco and alcohol consumption, nutrition, health, medications, sleep disturbance, life events, and attitudes but no items even remotely related to the suicidality probes found in instruments like the Zung Self-Rating Depression Scale (Zung, 1985) or the Hamilton Depression Rating Scale (Hamilton, 1960).

INFERENCES FROM THE DOMAINS OF PERSONALITY AND NEUROPSYCHOLOGY

Attempts to capture the personality of older suicide attempters have remained largely unsuccessful over more than 30 years of effort (Weissman, 1974). Studies of younger adults suggest a profile of hostility and impulsiveness (Coccaro et al., 1989). However, the variability of personality assessment, the problem of state versus trait, and the influence of cohort effects and gender in late life make it difficult to generalize adolescent and younger adult findings to the elderly. Batchelor and Napier (1953), in one of the rare reports on personality characteristics of older suicide attempters, found them seclusive and hypochondriacal, with restricted social interests. Pathological jealousy and suspiciousness were observed in some instances, but overall, individuals in the sample were categorized as either inadequate or vulnerable suggesting a psychological frailty and constriction. Neuroticism may also be characteristic of suicidal persons (Costa, 1991).

Neuropsychological investigations of suicide attempters also describe a constriction in executive thought, function as reflected in planning and problem solving (Weishaar & Beck, 1990). However, the contribution of impairments in executive function to the psychology of late-life suicide remains to be extracted from the confounding influence of character and affect that have been the more traditional focus of study.

WHERE ARE THE INTERVENTION STUDIES?

In 1988, the American Association of Retired Persons conducted a national survey of prevention and intervention programs for suicidal elderly (Mercer, 1989). Findings confirmed earlier assertions by Miller (1978) and McIntosh (1985) that direct, organized clinical efforts were rare in the extreme. Educational offerings for the professions and public at large, case finding, and legislative action were all minimal to nonexistent. Existing programs for the suicidal adults showed a general lack of emphasis on the problems of the elderly despite a recognition of a sizable problem. A number of model programs were cited that recognize the interrelations of the social, medical, and mental health determinants of late-life suicide. Aggressive and at times unconventional outreach for case finding, integration of programs across the array of social agencies and health care entities, education and training of new and existing personnel, and appropriate interventions including peer support and follow-through were identified as essential elements of effective programs. But even these systematic programs were barely in the beginning stages. The Seattle "gatekeepers" program is one such model effort that claims a reduction in suicides (Goldstein et al., 1993).

Although intervention studies for late-life suicide are few, there has been considerable work on reducing suicides across all age ranges through efforts that have little to do with traditional mental health systems. These include the reduction of carbon monoxide from coal gas, the reduction in prescriptions of barbiturates, the introduction of antidepressants with less toxicity in the event of overdose, and efforts to reduce the possession of handguns. Sadly, the development of suicide counseling centers and the growth in the number and utilization of antidepressants have not been accompanied by a reduction in elderly suicide rates (Brown, 1979). No more than 4% of calls to suicide hotlines are from the elderly (Osgood, 1992). The development of profiles describing high-risk populations has also had little effect on suicidal death. The problem of suicide across the life span is in part responsible for the development of the National Center for Injury Prevention and Control at the Centers for Disease Control (Shaffer, 1993).

In a novel approach, the American Association of Retired Persons will send two hundred volunteers to alert primary care physicians to the risk of late-life suicide (B. Davis, personal communication, December 10, 1992). Because 80% of older adults have attended religious services in the last month, a similar effort might be worth considering for the clergy. However, it is only in the past 5 years that mental health instruction has been introduced into the curriculum at a majority of seminaries. Most clergy with congregations have no training in the recognition and referral of individuals with mental illness (Clark, 1992). Nonetheless, just as the schools have become the base for programs to counter teenage suicide, religious institutions seem a reasonable choice for reaching senior citizens.

CONCLUSION

Suicidal behavior in early life is often impulsive. It is associated with female gender, active rather than passive self-injury, a family history of suicide, and a personal history of repeated suicidal ideas, substance abuse, and mental illness, particularly affective and anxiety disorders. In contrast, late-life suicidality is more often premeditated. It is characterized by male gender, social isolation, physical illness, disability, and fewer attempts, with more lethal methods and outcomes. Available information from younger clinical populations, epidemiological, and biological studies are not adequate to design preventive services. And the most recent estimates indicate that present mental health and social services that should reduce the associated morbidity and mortality are failing.

The lack of specialized intervention programs and a near absence of outcome studies reflect both the infrequency of suicide as well as the antagonism between the social and psychopathological theories of etiology. However, this antagonism may indicate as much about desirable interventions as it does about the lack of agreement. Any effective understanding about the causes and prevention of elderly suicide must address both social pathology and psychopathology. Reports of physician-assisted suicides (Altman, 1991) make the need for both theoretical and empirical data all the more urgent.

REFERENCES

Altman, L. K. (1991, July 27). Jury declines to indict a doctor who said he aided in a suicide. *New York Times,* p. 1.

Angell, M. (1990). Prisoners of technology: The case of Nancy Cruzan. *New England Journal of Medicine, 322,* 1226–1228.

Atchley, R. C. (1980). *Social forces in later life.* Belmont, CA: Wadsworth.

Bakken, E. (1991, January). Promoting public awareness of effective treatments for mental illness. *Psychiatric Times,* pp. 28–32.

Barr, W. B. (1992, December 10). Remarks at the *Too Young to Die* Conference on the National Suicide Survey conducted by Empire Blue Cross and Blue Shield and the Gallup Organization, Inc. New York, NY.

Barraclough, B. (1971). Suicide in the elderly. In D. W. K. Kay & A. Walks (Eds.), *Recent developments in psychogeriatrics* (pp. 87–97). Headly, U.K.: Royal Medico Psychological Association.

Batchelor, I. R. C., & Napier, M. B. (1953). Attempted suicide in old age. *British Medical Journal, 2,* 1186–1190.

Beck, A. T., Steer, R. A., Kovacs, M., & Garrison, B. (1985). Hopelessness and eventual suicide: A 10-year prospective study of patients hospitalized with suicidal ideation. *American Journal of Psychiatry, 142,* 559–563.

Blazer, D. G., Bachar, J. R., & Manton, K. G. (1986). Suicide in late life: Review and commentary. *Journal of the American Geriatrics Society, 34,* 519–525.

Brody, H. (1992). Assisted death—A compassionate response to a medical failure. *New England Journal of Medicine, 327,* 1384–1388.

Bron, B., Strack, M., & Rudolph, G. (1991). Childhood experiences of loss and suicide attempts: Significance in depressive states of major depressed and dysthymic or adjustment disordered patients. *Journal of Affective Disorders, 23,* 165–172.

Brown, J. H. (1979). Suicide in Britain: More attempts, fewer deaths, lessons for public policy. *Archives of General Psychiatry, 36,* 1119–1124.

Brown, T. R., & Sherman, T. J. (1972). Suicide prediction: A review. *Life Threatening Behavior, 2,* 67–98.

Clark, D. C. (1992, December 10). Remarks at the *Too Young to Die* Conference on the National Suicide Survey conducted by Empire Blue Cross and Blue Shield and the Gallup Organization, Inc. New York, NY.

Clayton, P. J. (1985). Suicide. *Psychiatric Clinics of North America, 8,* 203–214.

Coccaro, E. F., Siever, L. J., Klar, H. M., Mauer, G., Cochrane, K., Cooper, T. B., Mohs, R. C., & Davis, K. L. (1989). Serotonergic studies in patients with affective and personality disorders. *Archives of General Psychiatry, 46,* 587–599.

Conwell, Y., Caine, E. D., & Olsen, K. (1990). Suicide and cancer in late life. *Hospital and Community Psychiatry, 41,* 1334–1339.

Conwell, Y., Melanie, R., & Caine, E. D. (1990). Completed suicide at age 50 and over. *Journal of the American Geriatric Society, 38,* 640–644.

Cornoni-Huntley, J., Brock, D. B., Ostfeld, A. M., Taylor, J. O., & Wallace, R. B. (Eds.). (1986). Established populations for the Epidemiologic Studies of the Elderly resource data book (NIH Publication No. 86-2443). Washington, DC: U.S. Department of Health and Human Services.

Costa, P. T. (1991). Depression as an enduring disposition. In *Program and Abstracts* (p. 45). NIMH Consensus Development Conference on the Diagnosis and Treatment of Depression in Late Life, Bethesda, MD.

Cummings, E., & Henry, N. E. (1961). *Growing old: The process of disengagement.* New York: Basic Books.

Durkheim, E. (1951). *Suicide.* New York: Free Press. (Original work published 1891)

Dyer, E. R. (1992, December 10). Remarks at the *Too Young to Die* Conference on the National Suicide Survey conducted by Empire Blue Cross and Blue Shield and the Gallup Organization, Inc. New York, NY.

Easterlin, R. A. (1986). *The Easterlin Hypothesis,* (pp. 22–32). London: MacMillan Press.

Etzersdorfer, E., Sonnek, G., & Nagel-Kuess, S. (1992). Newspaper reports and suicide [To the editor]. *New England Journal of Medicine, 327,* 502–503.

Gallup, G. H. (1992, December 10). Remarks at the *Too Young to Die* Conference on the National Suicide Survey conducted by Empire Blue Cross and Blue Shield and the Gallup Organization, Inc. New York, NY.

Gallup Organization. (1992). *Executive summary: Attitude and incidence of suicide among the elderly.* Princeton, NJ: Author.

Goldstein, M., Colenda, C. C., Kennedy, G. J., Van Dooren, H., Van Stone, W., Hay, D. P., & Sadavoy, J. (1993). *Models of geropsychiatric practice.* Washington, DC: American Psychiatric Press.

Green, S. M. (1981). Levels of hopelessness in the general population. *British Journal of Clinical Psychology, 20,* 11–14.

Gurland, B. J., & Cross, P. J. (1983). Suicide among the elderly. In M. K. Aronson, R. Bennet, & G. J. Gurland (Eds.), *The acting-out elderly* (pp. 48–55). New York: Hawthorn Press.

Haas, A. P., & Hendin, G. E. (1983). Suicide among older people: Projections for the future. *Suicide and Life-Threatening Behavior, 13,* 147–154.

Hamilton, M. (1960). A rating scale for depression. *Journal of Neurology, Neurosurgery, and Psychiatry, 23,* 56–62.

Hawton, K., & Fagg, J. (1990). Deliberate self-poisoning and self-injury in older people. *International Journal of Geriatric Psychiatry, 5,* 367–373.

Hemenway, D., Solnick, S. J., & Colditz, G. A. (1993). Smoking and suicide among nurses. *American Journal of Public Health, 83,* 249–251.

Hershfeld, R. M. A., & Klerman, G. L. (1979). Treatment of depression in the elderly. *Geriatrics, 127,* 51–57.

Hill, R. D., Gallager, D., Thompson, L. W., & Ishida, T. (1988). Hopelessness as a measure of suicidal intent in the depressed elderly. *Psychology and Aging, 3,* 230–232.

Holden, C. (1992). A new discipline probes suicide's multiple causes. *Science, 256,* 1761–1762.

Horton-Deutsch, S. L., Clark, D. C., & Farran, C. J. (1992). Chronic dyspnea and suicide in elderly men. *Hospital and Community Psychiatry, 43,* 1198–1203.

Humphrey, R. (1991). *Final exit.* New York: Dell.

Kellerman, A. L., Rivara, F. P., Somes, G., Reay, D. T., Francisco, J., Banton, J. G., Prodzinski, J., Flinger, C., & Hackman, B. B. (1992). Suicide in the home in relation to gun ownership. *New England Journal of Medicine, 327,* 467–472.

The Kevorkian cure: Death (Editorial). (1990, December 12). *New York Times,* A17.

Klerman, G. L., Lavori, P. W., Rice, J., Reich, T., Endicott, J., Andreasen, N. C., Keller, M. B., & Hirschfield, R. M. (1985). Birth-cohort trends in rates of major depression among relatives of patients with affective disorder. *Archives of General Psychiatry, 42,* 689–694.

Lindsey, J. (1986). Trends in self-poisoning in the elderly 1974–1983. *International Journal of Geriatric Psychiatry, 1,* 37–43.

Lindsey, J. (1991). Suicide in the elderly. *International Journal of Geriatric Psychiatry, 6,* 355–361.

Loebel, J. P., Loebel, J. S., Dager, S. R., Centerwall, B. S., & Reay, D. T. (1991). Anticipation of nursing home placement may be a precipitant of suicide among the elderly. *Journal of the American Geriatric Society, 39,* 407–408.

Mackensie, T. B., & Popkin, M. K. (1987). Suicide in the medical patient. *International Journal of Psychiatry in Medicine, 17,* 3–22.

Maris, R. W. (1969). *Social forces in urban suicide.* New York: Dorsey Press.

Marzuk, P. M., Leon, A. C., Tardiff, K., Morgan, E. B., Marina, S., & Mann, J. (1992). The effect of access to lethal methods of injury on suicide rates. *Archives of General Psychiatry, 49,* 451–458.

McCall, P. L. (1991). Adolescent and elderly white male suicide trends: Evidence of changing well-being? *Journals of Gerontology: Social Sciences, 46,* S43–51.

McIntosh, J. L. (1985). Suicide among the elderly: Levels and trends. *American Journal of Orthopsychiatry, 55,* 288–293.

McIntosh, J. L., & Santos, J. F. (1981). Suicide among minority elderly: A preliminary investigation. *Suicide and Life Threatening Behavior, 11*(3), 151–166.

Meehan, P. J., Saltzberg, L. E., & Sattin, R. W. (1991). Suicides among older United States residents: Epidemiologic characteristics and trends. *American Journal of Public Health, 81,* 1198–1200.

Mercer, S. O. (1989). Elder suicide: A national survey of prevention and intervention programs. Washington, DC: American Association of Retired Persons.

Merloo, J. (1968). Hidden suicide. In H. L. P. Resnick (Ed.), *Suicidal behaviors: Diagnosis and management* (pp. 45–59). Boston: Little, Brown.

Miller, M. (1978). Geriatric suicide: The Arizona study. *Gerontologist, 18,* 488–495.

Murphy, G. E., Wetzel, R. D., Robins, E., & McEvoy, L. (1992). Multiple risk factors predict suicide in alcoholism. *Archives of General Psychiatry, 49,* 459–463.

Murphy, G. K. (1977). Cancer and the coroner. *Journal of the American Medical Association, 237,* 786–788.

National Center for Health Statistics. (1990). *Vital statistics of the United States, 1988: Vol. II. Mortality, Part B.* (DHHS Publication No. PHS 90-1102). Washington, DC: U.S. Government Printing Office.

Nelson, F. L., & Farberow, N. L. (1977). Indirect suicide in the elderly chronically ill patient. In K. Achte & J. Lonnqvist (Eds.), *Suicides research* (pp. 125–139). Helsinki: Psychiatry Finnica.

Osgood, N. J. (1985). *Suicide in the elderly.* Rockville, MD: Aspen.

Osgood, N. J. (1989). Risk identification strategies outlines in elderly suicide. *Psychiatric Times, 5,*(10) 1.

Osgood, N. J. (1992, December 10). Remarks at the *Too Young to Die* Conference on the National Suicide Survey conducted by Empire Blue Cross and Blue Shield and the Gallup Organization, Inc. New York, NY.

Owens, J. (1990). Age and attempted suicide. *Acta Psychiatrica Scandinavia, 82,* 385–388.

Parkin, D., & Stengal, E. (1965). Incidence of suicide attempts in an urban community. *British Medical Journal, 2,* 133–140.

Pritchard, C. (1992). Changes in elderly suicides in the USA and the developed world 1974–87: Comparison with current homicide. *International Journal of Geriatric Psychiatry, 7,* 125–134.

Quill, T. E. (1991). Death and dignity: A case of individualized decision making. *New England Journal of Medicine, 324,* 691–694.

Quill, T. E., Cassel, C. K., & Meier, D. E. (1992). Care of the hopelessly ill: Proposed criteria for physician assisted suicide. *New England Journal of Medicine, 327,* 1380–1384.

Rosenberg, M. L., Eddy, D. M., Wolpert, R. C., & Broumas, E. P. (1989). Developing strategies to prevent youth suicide. In C. R. Pfeffer (Ed.), *Suicide among youth: Perspectives on risk and prevention* (pp. 203–225). Washington, DC: American Psychiatric Press.

Shaffer, D. (1993). Suicide: Risk factors and the public health. *American Journal of Public Health, 83,* 171–172.

Shneidman, E. S. (1963). Orientation towards death: A vital aspect of the study of lives. In R. White (Ed.), *The study of lives* (pp. 145–162). New York: Prentice Hall.

Sorenson, S. B. (1991). Suicide among the elderly: Issues facing public health. *American Journal of Public Health, 81,* 1109–1110.

Tolchin, M. (1989, July 19). When long life is too much: Suicide rates among the elderly. *New York Times,* p. A1.

van Praag, H. M., & Plutchik, R. (1985). An empirical study on the "cathartic effect" of attempted suicide. *Psychiatry Press, 16,* 123–130.

Weishaar, M. E., & Beck, A. T. (1990). Cognitive approaches to understanding and treating suicidal behavior. In S. J. Blumenthal & D. J. Kupfer, (Eds.), *Suicide over the life cycle: Risk factor assessment, and treatment of suicidal patients* (pp. 469–498). Washington DC: American Psychiatric Press.

Weissman, M. M. (1974). The epidemiology of suicide attempts, 1960 to 1971. *Archives of General Psychiatry, 30,* 737–746.

Weissman, M. R., Klerman, G. L., Markowitz, J. S., & Ouellette, R. (1989). Suicidal ideation and suicide attempts in panic disorder and attacks. *New England Journal of Medicine, 321,* 1209–1214.

Whanger, A. D. (1989). Inpatient treatment of the older psychiatric patient. In E. Busse & D. G. Blazer (Eds.), *Geriatric psychiatry* (pp. 593–634). Washington, DC: American Psychiatric Press.

Woodbury, M. A., Manton, K. G., & Blazer, D. G. (1988). Trends in U.S. suicide mortality rates 1968 to 1982: Race and sex differences in age, period and cohort components. *International Journal of Epidemiology, 17,* 356–362.

Zung, W. W. K. (1985). A self-rating depression scale. *Archives of General Psychiatry, 12,* 63–70.

2

The Epidemiology of Late-Life Depression

GARY J. KENNEDY

A number of factors complicate the epidemiology and public health import of late-life depression. The definition of conditions that will benefit from treatment, the detection of incident cases, and the application of effective services to reduce case prevalence remain highly problematic. These problems exist despite the availability of therapies to lessen the pain and disability of depression across the spectrum of severity.

DEFINITIONS

The prevalence of depressive symptoms increases with age but the prevalence of major depressive disorders declines. This apparent paradox arises out of differing traditions that define depression in the elderly as either a symptom, a disorder, or a geriatric syndrome characterized—like incontinence, falls, and frailty—by multiple etiologies and presentations. However, epidemiological data supporting these three definitions of depression are complementary rather than conflicting. A synthesis of information regarding the epidemiologies of depressive symptoms and depressive disorders is required to better understand the relevance of depression to the well-being of older adults as well as the need for mental health services in late life.

Prevalence figures for depressive disorders are based on a diagnostic consensus reflecting therapeutic indications for individuals most likely to benefit from established treatments. Obviously, depressive symptoms identify persons at risk for a depressive disorder. However, most older adults have depressive symptoms that either are not congruent with diagnostic categories or coexist with physical illness that confounds their diagnostic relevance. These individuals represent a larger population in potential need in whom the benefits of treatment are less certain. Finally, because of the reciprocal nature of depression and disability, viewing late-life depression as a geriatric syndrome points to the need for a combination of therapeutic approaches to return the older person to optimum function.

There is considerable argument as to whether mood disturbances should be seen as categorical (diagnostic) phenomena or as a dimension of mental illness. Three sets of observations support the dimensional argument. First, the major neurotransmitter systems, most notably serotonin, are implicated in the etiologies of affective and anxiety disorders as well as psychotic and nonpsychotic illness (van Praag et al., 1990). Second, antidepressants are effective in the treatment of both depressive and anxiety disorders but are not adequate alone for the treatment of psychotic depression. Third, the threshold criteria for depressive disorders in the *Diagnostic and Statistical Manual of Mental Disorders* (*DSM III-R, DSM-IV;* American Psychiatric Association, 1987, 1994) are based more on consensus than empiricism.

In an attempt to cluster symptoms into statistic-empirical rather than consensus-derived diagnostic categories, Blazer et al. (1989) identified a pure type depressive cluster found almost exclusively among older adults. Another cluster was almost identical to the *DSM-III-R* diagnosis of major depression with melancholia. A third old-age cluster consisted of depressed mood, psychomotor retardation, difficulty concentrating, constipation, and poor self-assessed health, yet few of the members met criteria for major depression or dysthymia. These data suggest that a minor depressive syndrome of late life characterized by impaired cognition and poor physical health existed among older individuals, and that *DSM* diagnoses neither capture nor displace members of the minor depression group.

DEPRESSIVE DISORDERS AMONG
OLDER COMMUNITY RESIDENTS

The Epidemiologic Catchment Area Program (ECA) identified mental disorders among community residents. The prevalence of major depressive disorder ranged by site from 0.1% to 0.5% among older men and 1.0% to 1.6% among older women (Myers, Weissman, et al., 1984). However, anxiety disorders (particularly agoraphobia among women) overshadowed the frequency of depression and ranged from 3.6% for older men to 6.8% for older women. Because the ECA program excluded individuals with bereavement and physical conditions that might confound the decision to prescribe antidepressants, the ECA results underestimate the prevalence of clinically relevant depression (Kermis, 1986). Thus the ECA data do not represent the population of all older adults but do provide convincing evidence that depression is remarkably infrequent in healthy, not demented senior Americans.

DEPRESSIVE SYMPTOMS AMONG
COMMUNITY RESIDENTS

Information from more representative populations of older community residents is available in the form of clinically significant levels of depressive symptoms rather than codified disorders. The most widely used symptom survey instrument is the Center for Epidemiologic Studies Depression (CES-D) Scale (Radloff, 1977). Compared with ECA measures, the CES-D sacrifices diagnostic specificity for clinical sensitivity. When the CES-D is employed, the prevalence of depressive symptoms ranges from a low of 9% in Iowa and the Piedmont area of North Carolina (Blazer, Burchett, Service, & George, 1991) to 19% across Alabama (Foelker & Shewchuk, 1992). Combining both symptom and diagnostic measures, Blazer, Hughes, and George (1989) found at least one symptom of depression in 25% of community elders, with mild dysphoria in 19%, dysthymia in 2%, major depression in 0.8%, and mixed depression with anxiety in 1.2%.

DEPRESSIVE SYMPTOMS AMONG
CLINICALLY DEFINED SAMPLES

Significant levels of depressive symptoms have been found among 30% to 50% of elderly medical outpatients (Katz, Curil, & Nemetz, 1988).

Among nonpsychiatric inpatients, Rapp, Parisi, and Walsh (1988) found that 30% showed clinically significant elevations on depressive symptoms scales and that 15% met *DSM* criteria for a depressive disorder. However, only 10% of the diagnosable patients were identified by their primary care physicians as needing treatment (Rapp, Parisi, & Wallace, 1991). Depressed older adults occupy close to 40% of acute psychiatric beds. These patients are distinguished from their younger peers by the presence of psychosis in nearly 50% of cases and the likelihood that electroconvulsive therapy (ECT) will be administered (Myers, Kalayum, & Mei-tal, 1984).

Up to 60% of patients develop a major depression within 6 months following a stroke. Antidepressant treatment with nortriptyline guided by therapeutic levels, reduces depression and dependency (Lipsey, Robinson, Pearlson, Rao, & Price, 1984). Depression tends to remit spontaneously without antidepressants between 1 and 2 years following the stroke but impedes physical rehabilitation (Parikh, Lipsey, Robinson, & Price, 1987). In Parkinson's disease, depression appears in 40% of individuals, half with major depression, half with dysthymia. Antidepressant treatment will ameliorate the depressed mood but may not dramatically reduce the motor disability. Electroconvulsive therapy may substantially improve the depression but any gains in motor function will be transitory (Cummings, 1992). Depressive disorders appear to be frequent in persons with Alzheimer's (Lazarus, Newton, Cohler, Lesser, & Schweon, 1987; Rovner, Broadhead, Spencer, Carson, & Folstein, 1989) and multi-infarct disease but the prevalence of depression in representative as opposed to volunteer samples of individuals with dementia remains unclear.

RESIDENTIAL HEALTH CARE FACILITIES

The majority of nursing home residents experience a major mental illness (Goldfarb, 1962) with dementia, depression, and dementia complicated by depression being the most frequent disorders (Rovner, German, Broadhead, Moriss, & Brant, 1990). About 30% to 50% of older nursing home residents voice at least some depressive symptoms. The prevalence of major depressive disorder ranges from 6% to 25% (Katz & Parmelee, 1994), and the 6-month incidence following admission approaches 14% (Katz, Lesher, Kleban, Jethaanadani, & Parmelee, 1989). There are few controlled studies of antidepressant or the psychotherapeutic treatment of depression in nursing homes. Parmelee, Katz, and Lawton (in press) found that more than 40% of cases with major depression and more than 50% with minor depression remain symptomatic despite aggressive efforts at treatment.

DEPRESSION AMONG CAREGIVERS
OF RELATIVES WITH DEMENTIA

To find predictors of institutionalization, researchers have focused considerable attention on depression among caregivers of demented community residents (Cohen & Eisdorfer, 1988; Zarit, Peterson, & Bach-Peterson, 1980). Gallagher, Rose, Rivera, Losett, and Thompson (1989) found major depression in 46% of caregivers seeking help and in 18% of those not actively seeking assistance. Moreover, caregiver depression is not necessarily relieved by nursing home admission (Kiecolt-Gleser, Dura, Speicher, & Trask, 1991; Light & Lebowitz, 1989). Difficulties with separation-individuation or "letting go" add to the burden of caregiving (Gwyther, 1990), which has been compared with the experience of military wives whose husbands were declared missing in action (Boss, Caron, Horbal, & Mortomer, 1990).

OTHER FACTORS AFFECTING PREVALENCE

Low income, life events, and lack of opportunities for, or difficulties with, companionship heighten the risk of depression (Lin & Ensel, 1984; Ohara, Kohout, & Wallace, 1985; Phifer & Murrell, 1986). Older adults may also be more likely than younger adults to develop a major depressive episode following bereavement (Zisook, 1991). Measures of ethnicity and religious practice have also been related to depression, with community residents who identified themselves as Jewish having twice the prevalence of depressive symptoms as those identified as Catholic. Lack of attendance at religious services was associated with depression among the Catholics but not the Jews (Kennedy, Kelman, Thomas, Wisniewski, & Metz, 1987).

Although personality remains fairly stable from mid to late life (Hagberg, Samuelson, Lindberg, & Dehlinm, 1991; Schaie & Willis, 1991), character trait differences between older men and women emerge in advanced age (McCrae, 1989). Men take on more traditionally feminine traits; women assume a more masculine profile. Aged men are much more likely to live with a spouse than are aged women because of differences in survival. However, the survival advantage women experience is accompanied by higher rates of disability and solitary living than among older men. Nonetheless, once corrected for disability and medical conditions, gender differences in service utilization disappear (Thomas & Kelman, 1990). These gender differences are pertinent to the higher rates of depression among older women compared with higher rates of suicide among older men (McCleary, Chew, Hellsten, & Flynn-Bransford, 1991).

Depression, aside from consideration as an illness, may also be seen as a personality trait within the domain of neuroticism. As a trait, depression may reach criteria for dysthymia, predispose the vulnerable individual to major depression, contribute to poor treatment response, or impede rehabilitation (Costa, 1991). "Double depression," the appearance of a major depressive episode with a background of prior dysthymia or chronic depression, is seen in as many as one third of patients presenting to clinic with a mood disorder (Keller & Shapiro, 1982).

DISABILITY AND THE DYNAMICS OF DEPRESSIVE SYMPTOMS

Roth and Kay (1956) were among the first to note the relation of poor health and physical disability to the onset of late-life depression. Subsequently, Gurland, Wilder, and Berkman (1988) described a reciprocal relationship between depressive disorders and disability relevant to both etiology and treatment of each. Health and disability play the predominant role in explaining the prevalence and dynamics of depressive symptoms in older community residents overshadowing the contribution of sociodemographic, life event, and interpersonal factors. Among 1,855 elderly community residents of the Norwood section of the Bronx, 17% showed a significant level of depressive symptoms. Twenty-four months later, depressive symptoms emerged in 9%, persisted from baseline in 6%, and remitted in 7% of the respondents. The persistence rate was somewhat less than 50%, the remission rate was somewhat more than 50%, and more than 75% of the respondents remained asymptomatic (Kennedy, Kelman, & Thomas, 1990; Kennedy et al., 1989).

The major characteristics distinguishing individuals who remained asymptomatic from those in whom depressive symptoms emerged were increasing disability and declining health. Declining health followed by advanced age distinguished those with persistent symptoms from those in whom symptoms remitted. Only improved health was associated with symptom remission.

Clinical studies of older adults with major depression have generally emanated from specialized, state-of-the-art treatment programs. However, the Norwood sample received routine health care with only 8% of the persistence and only 11% of the remission group reporting any exposure to mental health specialists (Kennedy, Kelman, & Thomas, 1991). Psychotropic treatment among the depressed group was more often symptomatic, with the use of hypnotics and antianxiety agents, rather than definitive, with the use of an antidepressant. Only 6% of the depressed group received an antidepressant following baseline. Thus depressive symptoms were relatively persistent in the context of routine care and fluctuated with changes in health and disability.

DYNAMICS OF DEPRESSIVE DISORDERS

The best available data suggest that major depression disorders more often have a lifelong course in which the prevention of recurrences rather than induction of a remission becomes the long-range clinical concern (Frank, 1991). Consensus terminology regarding the course of depressive illness during treatment is of relatively recent origin (Frank et al., 1993). The phases of treatment are divided into acute, continuation, and maintenance with remission, relapse, and recurrence being the analogous symptom descriptors. Acute phase treatment brings an initial remission of symptoms followed by continuation therapy over the next 6 to 9 months to prevent relapse, defined as incomplete resolution of the index episode. Therapy is then maintained beyond the first year to prevent a recurrent depressive episode.

Present opinion regarding recovery among older adults hospitalized for a depressive episode is pessimistic (Burvil, Stampfer, & Hall, 1991; Murphy, 1991). Although two thirds recover, from one quarter to one third either remain relatively symptomatic or significantly disabled. The rates of relapse and recurrence increase among the elderly. In some studies, psychosocial factors are associated with poor outcome but cognitive impairment and physical illness are more consistent predictors. Placebo is inferior to both psychotherapy and antidepressants in inducing remission. Medication is superior to psychotherapy and placebo in preventing recurrence (Rush, 1991).

Data specifying the most effective pharmacological means to prevent recurrence are limited. Reducing the acute phase antidepressant dose by 50% to 60% for maintenance is better than placebo, but nearly half those treated at the reduced level experience recurrence. Also, dose reduction may contribute to incomplete remission of an initial episode leading to a persistent depressive condition (Rohrbaugh, Sholoskas, & Giller, 1989). Maintaining treatment at acute phase levels will achieve a recurrence-free interval for 36 months in close to 80% of patients (Georgotas, McCue, Cooper, Nagachandran, & Chang, 1988; Glen, Johnson, & Shepherd, 1984; Prien et al., 1984). Maintenance treatment with ECT has gained recent support (Hay & Hay, 1990) and may offer higher rates of recovery.

DEPRESSION, ASSOCIATED MORBIDITY, AND SERVICES UTILIZATION

The total of ambulatory care services utilized by older adults (Thomas & Kelman, 1990) as well as their entrance and permanence of stay in nursing facilities (Kelman & Thomas, 1990) are related to depressive symptoms and cannot be accounted for simply by associated disability and the weight of medical conditions. The Medical Outcome Study by Wells et al. (1990) showed that depressed outpatients were consistently more physically and socially dysfunctional than their peers with chronic physical conditions. Only cardiovascular disease carried a greater disability. The disability of depression tended to amplify rather than displace the disability associated with chronic conditions, and most chronic physical conditions were less disabling than minor depression.

More important, when depression coexists with another illness, a significant part of the associated morbidity is in excess, or avoidable. As only one example, psychiatric interventions for elderly inpatients with hip fractures resulted in significant cost-offsets and reduction in morbidity as defined by nursing home placement (Strain et al., 1991).

MORTALITY

The association of depressive disorders with shortened survival has been observed in a number of clinically based samples (Black, Winokur, & Nasrallah, 1987; Kerr, Shapira, & Roth, 1969; Koenig, Shelp, Goli, & Cohen, 1989; Murphy, Smith, Lindesay, & Slattery, 1988), may be related to greater cardiovascular mortality (Rabins, Harvis, & Koven, 1985), and is not explained by greater rates of suicide. In contrast, studies of older community residents indicate that neither depressive symptoms (Thomas, Kelman, Kennedy, Ahn, &

Yang, 1992) nor depressive disorders (Fredman et al., 1989) are consistently predictive of mortality once age, gender, health, and disability are controlled. This is not to say that depressing events such as bereavement (Kaprio, Koskenvuo, & Rita, 1987) are not associated with mortality in late life, but rather that other factors overshadow the contribution of depression. Similarly, depressive symptoms (Ashby, Ames, & West, 1991) and depressive disorders (Rovner et al., 1991) have been linked to mortality in nursing homes. However, in a facility with a highly developed program of treatment for depression, the increase in mortality was fully explained by greater disability and physical illness among the depressed (Parmelee et al., in press).

ACCESS AND ACCEPTANCE OF MENTAL HEALTH SERVICES

Of elderly community residents with an acknowledged need for mental health services, one third receive none and one third are treated by mental health specialists. The final third are treated by primary care providers who use pharmacotherapy that tends to be symptomatic rather than definitive (Burns & Taube, 1990). Older adults are more likely to receive suboptimal antidepressant therapy and are more likely to have adverse reactions.

Older adults are less willing to accept a mental health referral because of the stigma of mental illness and biases about old age and the inadequacies of psychiatric care (Lasoski, 1986). When the detection of a mental illness eludes the primary care provider, case findings by social service agencies are also inadequate. Area agencies on aging and the mental health delivery systems lack systematic linkage (Lebowitz, Light, & Bailkey, 1987). Ultimately, only 5% of older adults who might benefit receive any form of mental health service. Neither the number nor the distribution of psychiatrists approaches the lower estimates of need (Eisenberg, 1992).

Changes in social policy introduced to enhance geriatric mental health services have not proved to be highly effective. The Medicare reforms introduced in the 1980s were intended to expand access to outpatient psychiatric care for older adults but have been largely blunted by cost-containment efforts introduced as the Resource Based Relative Value Scale. The Omnibus Budget Reduction Act of 1987 called for improvements in the psychosocial well-being of nursing home residents (U.S.

Health Care Financing Administration, 1989) provided no funds for mental health services (Gottlieb, 1990). Despite evidence that mental health care provided by primary care physicians may reduce inappropriate medical and surgical procedures, reimbursement for psychotherapy remains inadequate.

CONCLUSION

Advances in the epidemiology of late-life depression have been accompanied by a near golden age of safe, effective antidepressants and psychotherapies. This wealth of treatment is countered by a poverty of application despite reforms in mental health care reimbursements, nursing home regulations, and the emergence of psychogeriatrics as a recognized subspecialty in the United States. The failed promise of better mental health in late life through gains in clinical science and enlightened public policy is nowhere more evident than in the increasing rates of late-life suicide.

REFERENCES

American Psychiatric Association. (1987, 1994). *The diagnostic and statistical manual of mental disorders* (3rd ed. rev., 4th ed.). Washington, DC: Author.

Ashby, D., Ames, D., & West, C. R. (1991). Psychiatric morbidity as prediction of mortality for residents of local authority homes for the elderly. *International Journal of Geriatric Psychiatry, 6,* 567–575.

Black, D. W., Winokur, G., & Nasrallah, A. (1987). Is death from natural causes still excessive in psychiatric patients? A follow-up of 1,593 patients with major affective disorder. *Journal of Nervous and Mental Disease, 175,* 674–689.

Blazer, D., Burchett, B., Service, C., & George, L. K. (1991). The association of age and depression among the elderly: An epidemiologic exploration. *Journals of Gerontology: Medical Sciences,* M210–215.

Blazer, D., Hughes, D. C., & George, L. K. (1989). The epidemiology of depression in an elderly community population. *Gerontologist, 27,* 281–287.

Blazer, D., Woodbury, M., Hughes, D. C., George, L. K., Manton, K. G., Bachar, J. R., Fowler, N., & Cohen, H. J. (1989). A statistical analysis of the classification of depression in a mixed community and clinical sample. *Journal of Affective Disorders, 16,* 11–20.

Boss, P., Caron, W., Horbal, J., & Mortomer, J. (1990). Predictors of depression in caregivers of dementia patients: Boundary ambiguity and mastery. *Family Process, 29,* 245–254.

Burns, B. J., & Taube, C. A. (1990). Mental health services in general medical care and nursing homes. In B. Fogel, A. Furino, & G. Gottlieb (Eds.), *Mental Health Policy for Older Americans* (pp. 63–83). Washington, DC: American Psychiatric Press.

Burvil, P. W., Stampfer, H. G., & Hall, W. D. (1991). Issues in the assessment of outcome in depressive illness in the elderly. *International Journal of Geriatric Psychiatry, 6,* 269–278.

Cohen, D., & Eisdorfer, C. (1988). Depression in family members caring for a relative with Alzheimer's disease. *Journal of the American Geriatrics Society, 36,* 885–889.

Costa, P. T. (1991). Depression as an enduring disposition. In *Program and Abstracts* (p. 45). NIMH Consensus Development Conference on the Diagnosis and Treatment of Depression in Late Life, Bethesda, MD.

Cummings, J. L. (1992). Depression in Parkinson's disease: A review. *American Journal of Psychiatry, 149,* 443–445.

Eisenberg, L. (1992). Sounding Board. Treating depression and anxiety in primary care—Closing the gap between knowledge and practice. *New England Journal of Medicine, 326,* 1080–1083.

Foelker, G. A., & Shewchuk, R. M. (1992). Somatic components and the CES-D. *Journal of the American Geriatrics Society, 40,* 259–262.

Frank, E. (1991). Long-term prevention of recurrence in the elderly. In *Program and Abstracts* (pp. 77–79). NIMH Consensus Development Conference on the Diagnosis and Treatment of Depression in Late Life, Bethesda, MD.

Frank, E., Prien, R. F., Jarret, R. B., Keller, M. B., Kupfer, D. J., Lavoir, P., Rush, A. J., & Weissman, M. M. (1991). Conceptualization and rationale for consensus definitions of terms in major depressive disorder: Response, recovery, remission, relapse and recurrence. *Archives of General Psychiatry, 48,* 851–855.

Fredman, L., Schoenbach, V., Kaplan, B. H., Blazer, D. G., James, S. A., Kleinbaum, D. G., & Yankaskas, B. (1989). The association between depressive symptoms and mortality among older participants in the Epidemiologic Catchment Area-Piedmont Health Survey. *Journal of Gerontology: Social Sciences, 44,* S149–156.

Gallagher, D., Rose, J., Rivera, P., Losett, S., & Thompson, L. W. (1989). Prevalence of depression in family caregivers. *Gerontologist, 29,* 449–456.

Georgotas, A., McCue, R. E., Cooper, T. B., Nagachandran, N., & Chang, I. (1988). How effective and safe is continuation therapy in elderly depressed patients? *Archives of General Psychiatry, 45,* 929–932.

Glen, A. I. M., Johnson, A. L., & Shepherd, M. (1984). Continuation therapy with lithium and amitriptyline in unipolar depressive illness: A randomized, double-blind, controlled trial. *Psychological Medicine, 14,* 37–50.

Goldfarb, A. I. (1962). Prevalence of psychiatric disorders in metropolitan old age and nursing homes. *Journal of the American Geriatric Society, 10,* 77–84.

Gottlieb, G. L. (1990). Market segmentation. In B. S. Fogel, A. Furino, & G. L. Gottlieb (Eds.), *Mental health policy for older Americans: Protecting minds at risk* (pp. 135–156). Washington, DC: American Psychiatric Press.

Gurland, B. J., Wilder, D. E., & Berkman, C. (1988). Depression and disability in the elderly: Reciprocal relations and changes with age. *International Journal of Geriatric Psychiatry, 3,* 163–179.

Gwyther, L. P. (1990). Letting go: Separation-individuation in a wife of an Alzheimer's patient. *Gerontologist, 30,* 698–702.

Hagberg, B., Samuelson, G., Lindberg, B., & Dehlinm, O. (1991). Stability and change of personality in old age and its relation to survival. *Journals of Gerontology: Psychological Sciences, 46,* 285–291.

Hay, D., & Hay, L. (1990). The role of ECT in the treatment of depression. In C. D. McCann & N. S. Endler (Eds.), *Depression: New directions in theory, research, and practice* (pp. 255–272). Toronto: Wall & Emerson.

Kaprio, J., Koskenvuo, M., & Rita, H. (1987). Mortality after bereavement: A prospective study of 95,647 widowed persons. *American Journal of Public Health, 77,* 283–287.

Katz, I. R., Curil, S., & Nemetz, A. (1988). Functional psychiatric disorders in the elderly. In L. W. Lazarus (Ed.), *Essentials of geriatric psychiatry* (pp. 113–137). New York: Springer.

Katz, I. R., Lesher, E., Kleban, M., Jethaanadani, V., & Parmelee, P. (1989). Clinical features of depression in the nursing home. *International Psychogeriatrics, 1,* 5–15.

Katz, I. R., & Parmelee, P. A. (1994). Depression in elderly patients in the residential care settings. *Diagnosis and treatment of depression in late life* (pp. 437–462). Washington, DC: American Psychiatric Press.

Keller, M. B., & Shapiro, R. W. (1982). "Double depression": Superimposition of acute depressive episodes on chronic depressive disorders. *American Journal of Psychiatry, 139,* 438–442.

Kelman, H. R., & Thomas, C. (1990). Transitions between community and nursing home residence in an urban elderly population. *Journal of Community Health, 15,* 105–122.

Kennedy, G. J., Kelman, H. R., & Thomas, C. (1990). The emergence of depressive symptoms in late life: The importance of declining health and increasing disability. *Journal of Community Health, 15,* 93–104.

Kennedy, G. J., Kelman, H. R., & Thomas, C. (1991). Persistence and remission of depressive symptoms in late life. *American Journal of Psychiatry, 148,* 174–178.

Kennedy, G. J., Kelman, H. R., Thomas, C., Wisniewski, W., & Metz, H. (1987). Religious preference, attendance at services and the prevalence of depressive symptoms in the elderly. *Gerontologist, 27,* 260A.

Kennedy, G. J., Kelman, H. R., Thomas, C., Wisniewski, W., Metz, H., & Bijur, P. (1989). Hierarchy of characteristics associated with depressive symptoms in an urban elderly sample. *American Journal of Psychiatry, 146,* 220–225.

Kermis, M. D. (1986). The epidemiology of mental disorders in the elderly: A response to the Senate/AARP report. *Gerontologist, 26,* 482–487.

Kerr, T. A., Shapira, K., & Roth, M. (1969). The relationship between premature death and affective disorders. *British Journal of Psychiatry, 115,* 1277–1282.

Kiecolt-Gleser, J. K., Dura, J. R., Speicher, C. E., & Trask, O. J. (1991). Spousal caregivers of dementia victims: Longitudinal changes in immunity and health. *Psychosomatic Medicine, 53,* 345–362.

Koenig, H. G., Shelp, F., Goli, V., & Cohen, H. J. (1989). Survival and health care utilization among elderly medical inpatients with major depression. *Journal of the American Geriatrics Society, 37,* 599–606.

Lasoski, M. C. (1986). Reasons for low utilization of mental health services by the elderly. In T. L. Brink (Ed.), *Clinical gerontology: A guide to assessment and intervention* (pp. 1–18). Binghamton, NY: Haworth Press.

Lazarus, L. W., Newton, N., Cohler, B., Lesser, J., & Schweon, C. (1987). Frequency and presentation of depressive symptoms in patients with primary degenerative dementia. *American Journal of Psychiatry, 144,* 41–45.

Lebowitz, B. D., Light, E., & Bailkey, F. (1987). Mental health center services for the elderly: The impact of coordination with area agencies on aging. *Gerontologist, 27,* 699–702.

Light, E., & Lebowitz, B. D. (1989). *Alzheimer's disease treatment and family stress: Directions for research.* Rockville, MD: National Institute of Mental Health.

Lin, N., & Ensel, W. M. (1984). Depression mobility and its social etiology: The role of life events and social support. *Journal of Health and Social Behavior, 25,* 176–188.

Lipsey, J. R., Robinson, R. G., Pearlson, G. D., Rao, K., & Price, T. R. (1984). Nortriptyline treatment of post-stroke depression. A double blind study. *Lancet, 1*(8372), 297–300.

McCleary, R., Chew, K. S. Y., Hellsten, J. J., & Flynn-Bransford, M. (1991). Age- and sex-specific cycles in United States suicides, 1973 to 1985. *American Journal of Public Health, 81,* 1494–1497.

McCrae, R. R. (1989). Age differences and changes in the use of coping mechanisms. *Journals of Gerontology: Psychological Sciences, 44,* 161–169.

Murphy, E. (1991). The course of depression in late life. In *Program and Abstracts* (pp. 31–33). NIMH Consensus Development Conference on the Diagnosis and Treatment of Depression in Late Life, Bethesda, MD.

Murphy, E., Smith, R., Lindesay, J., & Slattery, J. (1988). Increased mortality rates in late-life depression. *British Journal of Psychiatry, 152,* 347–353.

Myers, J. K., Kalayum, B., & Mei-tal, V. (1984). Late-onset delusional depression: A distinct clinical entity? *Journal of Clinical Psychiatry, 45,* 347–349.

Myers, J. K., Weissman, M. M., Tischler, G. L., Holzer, C. E., Leat, P. J., Orvaschel, H., Anthony, J. C., Boyd, J. H., Burke, J. D., Kramer, M., & Stoltzman, R. (1984). Six month prevalence of psychiatric disorders in the community. *Archives of General Psychiatry, 41,* 959–967.

Ohara, M. W., Kohout, F. J., & Wallace, R. B. (1985). Depression among the rural elderly. *Journal of Nervous and Mental Disease, 173,* 582–589.

Parikh, R. M., Lipsey, J. R., Robinson, R. G., & Price, T. R. (1987). Two-year longitudinal study of post-stroke mood disorders: Dynamic changes in correlates of depression at one and two years. *Stroke, 18,* 579–584.

Parmelee, P., Katz, I. R., & Lawton, M. P. (in press). Depression and mortality among institutionalized aged. *Journal of Gerontology.*

Phifer, J. F., & Murrell, S. A. (1986). Etiologic factors in the onset of depressive symptoms in older adults. *Journal of Abnormal Psychology, 95,* 282–291.

Prien, R. F., Kupfer, D. J., Mansky, O. A., Small, J. G., Tuason, V. B., Voss, C. B., & Johnson, W. E. (1984). Drug therapy in the prevention of recurrences in unipolar and bipolar affective disorders: A report of the NIMH Collaborative Study Group comparing lithium carbonate, imipramine, and a lithium carbonate-imipramine combination. *Archives of General Psychiatry, 41,* 1096–1104.

Rabins, P. V., Harvis, K., & Koven, S. (1985). High fatality rates of late-life depression associated with cardiovascular disease. *Journal of Affective Disorders, 9,* 165–167.

Radloff, L. (1977). The CES-D Scale: A self report depression scale for research in the general population. *Applied Psychological Measurement, 1,* 385–406.

Rapp, S. R., Parisi, S., & Wallace, C. E. (1991). Comorbid psychiatric disorders in elderly medical patients; A 1 year prospective study. *Journal of the American Geriatrics Society, 39,* 124–141.

Rapp, S. R., Parisi, S. A., & Walsh, D. A. (1988). Psychologic dysfunction and physical health among elderly medical inpatients. *Journal of Consulting and Clinical Psychology, 56,* 851–855.

Rohrbaugh, R. M., Sholoskas, D. E., & Giller, E. L., Jr. (1989). Lifetime course of chronic depression in older men. *Journal of Geriatric Psychiatry and Neurology, 2,* 89–95.

Roth, M., & Kay, D. W. K. (1956). Affective disorder arising in the senium, II: Physical disability as an aetiologic factor. *Journal of Mental Science, 102,* 141–150.

Rovner, B. W., Broadhead, J., Spencer, M., Carson, K., & Folstein, M. F. (1989). Depression and Alzheimer's disease. *American Journal of Psychiatry, 146,* 350–353.

Rovner, B. W., German, P. S., Brant, L. J., Clark, R., Burton, L., & Folstein, M. F. (1991). Depression and mortality in nursing homes. *Journal of the American Medical Association, 265,* 993–996.

Rovner, B. W., German, P. S., Broadhead, J., Morriss, R. K., & Brant, L. J. (1990). The prevalence and management of dementia and other psychiatric disorders in nursing homes. *International Psychogeriatrics, 2,* 13–24.

Rush, A. J. (1991). Overview of treatment options in the depressed elderly. In *Program and Abstracts* (pp. 46–48). NIMH Consensus Development Conference on the Diagnosis and Treatment of Depression in Late Life, Bethesda, MD.

Schaie, K. W., & Willis, S. L. (1991). Adult personality and psychological performance: Cross-sectional and longitudinal analyses. *Journal of Gerontology: Psychological Sciences, 46,* 275–284.

Strain, J. J., Lyons, J. S., Hammer, J. S., Fahs, M., Lebovits, A., Paddison, P. L., Snyder, S., Strauss, E., Burton, R., & Nuber, G. (1991). Cost offset from a psychiatric consultation-liaison intervention with elderly hip fracture patients. *American Journal of Psychiatry, 148,* 1004–1049.

Thomas, C., & Kelman, H. R. (1990). Health services use among the elderly under alternative health service delivery systems. *Journal of Community Health, 15,* 77–92.

Thomas, C., Kelman, H. R., Kennedy, G. J., Ahn, C., & Yang, C-y. (1992). Depressive symptoms and mortality in the elderly 1992. *Journals of Gerontology: Social Sciences, 47,* S80–87.

U.S. Health Care Financing Administration. (1989). Medicare and Medicaid; Requirements for long-term care facilities: Final rule with request for comments. *Federal Register, 54,* 5316–5337.

van Praag, H. M., Asnis, G. M., Kahn, R. S., Brown, S. L., Korn, M., Friedman, J. M., & Wetzler, S. (1990). Monoamines and abnormal behavior: A multi-aminergic perspective. *British Journal of Psychiatry, 157,* 723–734.

Wells, K. B., Stewart, A., Hays, R. D., Burnam, M. A., Rogers, W., Daniels, M., Berry, S., Greenfield, S., & Ware, J. (1990). The functioning and well-being of depressed patients: Results from the Medical Outcomes Study. *Journal of the American Medical Association, 263*(5), 659–660.

Zarit, S., Peterson, K., & Bach-Peterson, J. (1980). Relatives of impaired elderly: Correlates of feelings of burden. *Gerontologist, 20,* 649–655.

Zisook, A. (1991). Diagnostic and treatment considerations in depression associated with late life bereavement. In *Program and Abstracts* (pp. 88–90). NIMH Consensus Development Conference on the Diagnosis and Treatment of Depression in Late Life, Bethesda, MD.

3

Biological Commonalities among Aging, Depression, and Suicidal Behavior

LON S. SCHNEIDER

Suicidal behavior or depression among the elderly may arise from a combination of genetic factors, developmental experiences, social relationships, stress, psychopathology, physical illness, and neurobiology. As discussed in other chapters of this volume, the timing of a suicidal act is related to environmental or state-dependent factors such as stress, loss, or depression. However, the vulnerability that an individual might have to the thinking, planning, and completing of a suicidal act may be determined more by enduring or "trait" factors than by environmental stress or a depressive episode. Examples of such long-standing factors are early developmental experiences, personality, recurrent cognitive processes, and underlying neurobiological factors. Depending on one's perspective, these enduring factors are subject to greater or lesser degrees of change as a person ages.

It is conceivable that a "neurobiological vulnerability" to suicide might undergo modulation by age-related changes in neurobiological systems. To the degree that changes in particular neurotransmitter systems have been implicated in suicide and depression, the serotonin system and hypothalamic pituitary adrenal axis have received the most attention. Both have been imputed as state, strait, or vulnerability markers in mood disorder and in suicide.

This chapter will briefly review selected evidence for existence of common biological changes related to depression, suicide, as well as to aging itself.

BIOLOGICAL CHANGES IN AGING AND DEPRESSION

Many of the neurochemical changes associated with aging are at least superficially similar to changes that have been described with depression. For example, normal aging is associated with decreased brain concentrations of serotonin, dopamine, norepinephrine and their metabolites (HVA, 5-HIAA); increased brain MAO-B activity; increased hypothalamic-pituitary-adrenal (HPA) activity; and increased sympathetic nervous system activity. Yet, we have sparse data available in this area, and what we have is occasionally contradictory. For example, in normal aging, although brain serotonin concentrations decrease in some areas with aging, they are unchanged in others (Marcussen et al., 1987). On the other hand, the density of brain ^{3}H-imipramine receptors increases with age in some brain areas but not in others (Owen et al., 1986; Severson, 1986).

HYPOTHALAMIC-PITUITARY-ADRENAL AXIS IN DEPRESSION, SUICIDE, AND AGING

Depression in all age groups is associated with hyperactivity and dysregulation of the hypothalamic-pituitary-adrenal (HPA) axis. This is characterized, in part, by elevated plasma and urinary cortisol, increased corticotropin-releasing hormone (CRH), blunted corticotropin (ACTH) response to CRH, and by resistance of cortisol to suppression by dexamethasone. Indeed, increased cortisol secretion is probably the most consistently observed physiological abnormality in patients with major depression.

Total urinary-free cortisol may reliably distinguish depressed from nondepressed individuals in clinical studies. The levels of cortisol, furthermore, appear to correlate with the severity of depression, with the presence of psychotic features, and with cognitive impairment (Kellner, Rubinow, & Post, 1986). Anatomical imaging research shows correlations of cortisol with brain ventricular enlargement (Kellner, Rubinow, Gold, & Post, 1983) and with enlargement of the pituitary and adrenal glands (Rao et al., 1989).

The dexamethasone suppression test (DST) was intended to identify the cortisol dysregulation associated with melancholic major depression and, hence, to serve as a marker for the disorder (Carroll, Greden, & Feinberg, 1981). Aging itself is associated with increasing plasma cortisol levels, and postdexamethasone cortisol concentration is higher in older, healthy subjects than in younger (Weiner, Davis, Mohs, & Davis, 1987). Increased age among depressed patients is associated with increased cortisol nonsuppression (Alexopoulos et al., 1984; Carrol et al., 1981; Davis et al., 1984). For example, within a predominantly elderly depressed inpatient group, 86% of those over 72 years of age had a positive DST compared with 58% below that age (Alexopoulos et al., 1984).

Nevertheless, it is unclear whether DST nonsuppression is specifically associated with aging per se in normal subjects (Tourigny-Rivard, Raskind, & Rivard, 1981) or, possibly, with other factors such as dexamethasone dose, or age-related diminished urinary clearance of cortisol (American Psychiatric Association Task Force on Laboratory Tests in Psychiatry, 1987). Drugs that increase the metabolism or clearance of dexamethasone may cause false positive results and include sedatives, anticonvulsants, antidepressants, and alcohol. Many medical illnesses that are particularly prevalent among the elderly cause a positive DST, including diabetes mellitus; cardiac, renal, and hepatic disease; cancer; and dehydration.

Nonsuppression on the DST occurs in about 50% of hospitalized, depressed, mixed-age adult patients, but when outpatients and nonmelancholic major depression are considered, a positive DST fails to characterize most patients with depression. Factors associated with the failure to suppress dexamethasone in depressed patients include severity of depression, physical illness, medication, inpatient status, weight loss, and aging (American Psychiatric Association Task Force on Laboratory Tests in Psychiatry, 1987).

The DST is not generally specific for major depression and has been applied in a number of different clinical situations including mania, anorexia, and dementia. It has been advocated to be useful in distinguishing major depression from primary dementia, or dementia from "pseudodementia." But when these studies are critically reviewed, approximately one half of Alzheimer's disease subjects without depression have positive DSTs (Addonizio & Shamoian, 1986).

The failure of dexamethasone to suppress cortisol (or its rapid release from suppression) seems to be state dependent, tending to occur during a depressive episode. It may normalize early in the course of depression or treatment, even without clinical improvement, but it is not a useful predictor of illness course. Conversely, patients may clinically improve while maintaining a positive DST, but also may be at increased risk for relapse (Carroll, 1985).

It is likely that the sensitivity of the DST among an elderly population is greater than in a younger population (Alexopoulos et al., 1984), but at the expense of reduced specificity for depression. Within an already diagnosed elderly depressed group, a positive DST may identify those with relatively more severe symptoms or a poor prognosis. Because abnormal DSTs occur frequently in Alzheimer's disease, other dementia, and medical illness, it appears that the test has limited diagnostic value in discriminating these disorders from primary depression in the elderly.

HPA-axis dysregulation or a positive DST may be associated with suicide as well as with depression. Elevated urinary-free cortisol and hydroxycorticosteroids have been observed in both suicide attempters and completers (Bunney, Fawcett, Davis, & Gifford, 1969; Ostroff et al., 1982). Rapid release from dexamethasone suppression or a "positive" DST has been associated with increased likelihood of suicide (Targum, Rosen, & Capodanno, 1983), as has a failure of the DST to normalize during a depressive episode (Yerevanian et al., 1983). As mentioned earlier, CRH is hypersecreted from the hypothalamus in depression. A decreased density of CRH receptors in the frontal cortex of suicide victims has been reported, suggesting a down regulation because CRH levels are normal (Nemeroff, Owens, Bissette, Andorn, & Stanley, 1988). Similarly, increased CRH in the cerebrospinal fluid (CSF) of suicide victims has been reported (Arato et al., 1991).

Considering the fragmentary evidence, it is highly speculative to consider that aging, depression, and suicide may interact. Normal aging may be associated with enhanced limbic-hypothalamic-pituitary-adrenal-axis activity, possibly because of age-associated neuronal degeneration in the hippocampus. The neuronal degeneration in turn may result from increased levels of glucocorticoids associated with both depression and aging. Depressive illness in the elderly or repetitive stressful life events may exacerbate this process. It is even more speculative to consider that these elderly depressed may then have an increased risk for suicide, based on independent observations of decreased CRH receptors and a positive DST as associational factors for suicide.

SEROTONIN FUNCTION IN DEPRESSION, SUICIDE, AND AGING

Deficits in the serotonin neurotransmitter system have been implicated in major depression and in suicide. Many studies suggest that 5-hydroxyindole acetic acid (5-HIAA), a metabolite of serotonin, is decreased in the CSF of depressed patients, suggesting a reduced turnover of serotonin (e.g., Asberg, Nordstrom, & Traskman-Bendz, 1986). Pre- and postsynaptic serotonin function may be altered as well (Stanley & Mann, 1983; Stanley, Virgilio, & Gershon, 1982).

Among suicide victims, at least, there is evidence for a decrease in the number of presynaptic imipramine receptors (Stanley et al., 1982) and an increase in the number of postsynaptic 5-HT_2 receptors (Stanley & Mann, 1983). This latter finding may represent upregulation due to decreased intrasynaptic serotonin. With respect to aging and depression, however, there was limited clinical information on the depressive symptoms in these mixed-age adult suicide victims. An interesting finding is the observation of brain hemispheric asymmetry of imipramine binding density in younger adult suicide victims, which is said to be a reversal of the expected asymmetry (Arato et al., 1991).

The idea that the alteration in serotonin may be more related to suicide than to depression is supported by observations of increased 5-HT_2 receptor density in elderly depressed patients dying of natural causes (Severson, Marcussen, Osterburg, Finch, & Winblad, 1985). However, contradictory information also exists. For example, CSF 5-HIAA was not different in patients with a personal or family history of suicide (Roy-Byrne et al., 1983). In one study, only the concentration of 5-HIAA in the hippocampus was increased in suicide victims. The concentrations of serotonin and the densities of 5-HT_1, 5-HT_2, and imipramine binding sites did not differ from controls in another report (Owen et al., 1986).

Although there exists a modest literature evaluating CSF markers in mixed-aged depressed and suicidal patients, only one study has focused specifically on elderly depressed subjects. In this subject, both CSF

5-HIAA and HVA, a metabolite of dopamine, were lower in elderly depressed suicide attempters than in depressed nonsuicide attempters and controls (Jones et al., 1990).

PLATELET ³H-IMIPRAMINE BINDING DENSITY

Regional localization and other studies suggest that specific brain ^{3}H-imipramine binding sites are correlated with serotonin patterns of innervation and are located on presynaptic serotonergic nerve terminals (Langer et al., 1987; Severson, 1986). The active component for this binding site has a role in modulating neuronal serotonin uptake.

The ^{3}H-imipramine binding site is also found on platelets and shares many characteristics with the brain binding site. Although the precise function of the platelet receptor remains obscure, it also seems closely related to the presynaptic serotonin uptake site and may be considered a marker for serotonergic dysfunction. Studies of imipramine binding are useful, especially because serotonergic dysfunction may characterize a subgroup of major depression patients, perhaps those who are more suicidal, and since, in brain, this may be the relevant site of action for tricyclic antidepressants.

Thus, during the past decade, platelet ^{3}H-imipramine binding density (B_{max}) has been examined extensively as a biological marker for mood disorder. Approximately two thirds of the studies have reported B_{max} values that are reduced 10% to 54% in groups of depressed patients compared with controls. There are over 70 controlled, clinical studies involving various diagnostic classifications. Platelet imipramine binding density seems to be decreased in obsessive-compulsive disorder, anorexia, and enuresis, also. There may be a differential decrease in density among certain depressive subtypes (Baron et al., 1986; Lewis & McChesney, 1985), including those with a family history of depression (Lewis & McChesney, 1985; Schneider, Fredrickson, Severson, & Sloane, 1986). However, a well-designed multicenter study failed to find significant differences between mixed-age adult depressed and controls (Mellerup & Langer, 1990).

Elderly unipolar depressed patients also show a 20% to 42% decrease in binding density when they are compared with age-appropriate controls (Nemeroff, Knight, et al., 1988; Schneider, Severson, & Sloane, 1985; Suranyi-Cadotte et al., 1985) although, again, this is not always so (Georgotas, Schweitzer, McCue, Armour, & Friedhoff, 1987).

Differences among specific depression subtypes in the elderly have not been widely studied, although receptor density seems to be somewhat lower in elderly depressed compared with a younger depressed cohort (Nemeroff, Knight, et al., 1988). There is one report that platelet imipramine density may discriminate between depression secondary to medical illness and primary major depression in an elderly population, with B_{max} decreased in primary depression patients compared with secondary depression patients and with controls (Schneider, Severson, Sloan, et al., 1988).

The effect of age on platelet binding density has not been systematically investigated. A few studies, using either age correlations or younger and older age cohorts of depressed and nondepressed, suggest an increase, decrease, or ño change in density with age. Further limitations are that the age ranges in these studies have been restricted, not including patients older than about 65 years. Animal studies suggest brain binding sites increase with age (Severson, 1986). It is not known if the imipramine binding site represents a trait or a state characteristic. The evidence suggesting state dependence is that depressed patients treated with electroconvulsive therapy showed an increase in binding density (Langer, Sechter, Loo, Raisman, & Zarifian, 1986). The effects of various medications, including tricyclic antidepressants, and disease states on the imipramine site have not been well researched. But it is clear that serotonin uptake blockers such as fluoxetine, paroxetine, citalopram, and chlorimipramine affect imipramine binding values.

Overall, platelet ^{3}H-imipramine binding density does not seem to be affected in groups of Alzheimer's disease (AD) patients (Nemeroff, Knight, et al., 1988; Schneider, Severson, Chui, et al., 1988; Suranyi-Cadotte et al., 1985) compared with controls. But there is some evidence that AD patients with agitation and delusions have a lower density than AD patients without these symptoms (Schneider et al., 1988). With respect to suicide attempts, depressed patients who made violent attempts had significantly higher platelet imipramine binding density than patients who made attempts by nonviolent means (Wagner et al., 1987). This finding is in contrast to the decreased brain imipramine binding density of suicide victims discussed earlier.

In summary, serotonin function markers may be related to violence, depression, and suicide in young adults. In the elderly, the situation is less clear. Many findings are fragmentary and conflicting. There may be a different neurobiology in suicide attempters compared with completers.

CONCLUSION

The neurotransmitter systems implicated in early life suicide change with age such that one would expect that the neurobiological risk of suicide should be highest in late life. However, studies of late-life suicidal behavior tend to emphasize psychosocial and psychopathological risk factors. For instance, as discussed elsewhere in this volume, major risk factors for suicide in the elderly include male gender, Caucasian race, living alone, marital separation, recent interpersonal loss, concurrent physical illness, depressive disorder, and alcohol abuse. There are several reasons the contribution of neurobiological factors to late life risk of suicide appears less sizable than expected. First, the strength of psychosocial associations may far outweigh clinically the relatively subtle neurobiological risk factors for late-life suicide. Second, the relatively stronger psychosocial associations to suicide make the neurobiology of the phenomenon much harder to study scientifically. Third, it also seems reasonable that subjects at substantial neurobiological risk for suicide would have completed suicide earlier in life. Finally, the neurobiological factors for suicide in late life may be much different from those in younger groups or counterbalanced by as yet unknown neurohumoral changes in old age. Table 3–1 summarizes current findings regarding biological factors in elderly suicide.

As researchers continue their efforts in this field, extremely high risk groups such as elderly white males, aged 80 to 84 years, may provide an especially rich population for further study of neurobiological features of suicide. And their numbers are increasing almost as rapidly as the fastest growing group of elders, those 85 and older.

TABLE 3–1

Summary of Findings Regarding the Presence or Absence of Biological Commonalities between Aging, Depression, and Suicide

Biological Component	Advanced Age	Depression	Suicide
HPA axis dexamethasone suppression test	+	+	+
CSF 5-HIAA		?	↓
Brain ^{3}H-imipramine density	↑		↓ or nc
Brain 5-HT$_2$ density	?↑		↑ or nc
Platelet ^{3}H-imipramine binding	↑ or ↓	↓	?*

nc = no change; + = positive; ↑ = increased; ↓ = decreased.
* = increased in suicide attempters.

Methods of controlling for the contribution to suicide of psychosocial risk factors must be devised. With adequate control of psychosocial factors, differences between suicide completers and repeaters (those with multiple attempts) may be worthy of special attention in research. For example, repeaters may have high levels of CSF serotonin and 5-HIAA, and higher platelet 5-HT$_2$ factors. By comparison, completers may show decreased CSF 5-HIAA, decreased presynaptic ^{3}H-imipramine binding, and higher levels of cortisol.

REFERENCES

Addonizio, G., & Shamoian, C. A. (1986). Depression and dementia. In D. V. Jeste (Ed.), *Neuropsychiatric dementia* (pp. 73–109). Washington, DC: American Psychiatric Press.

Alexopoulos, G. S., Young, R. L., Kocsis, J. H., Brockner, N., Butler, T. A., & Stokes, P. E. (1984). Dexamethasone suppression test in geriatric depression. *Biological Psychiatry, 19,* 1567–1571.

American Psychiatric Association Task Force on Laboratory Tests in Psychiatry. (1987). The dexamethasone suppression test: An overview of its current status in psychiatry. *American Journal of Psychiatry, 144,* 1253–1262.

Arato, M., Tekes, K., Tothfalusi, L., Magyer, K., Palkovits, M., Frecska, E., Falus, A., & MacCrimmon, D. J. (1991). Reversed hemispheric asymmetry of imipramine binding in suicide victims. *Biological Psychiatry, 29,* 699–702.

Asberg, M., Nordstrom, P., & Traskman-Bendz, L. (1986). Cerebrospinal fluid studies in suicide: An overview. In J. J. Mann & M. Stanley (Eds.), *Psychobiology of suicide behavior* (pp. 76–95). New York: New York Academy of Sciences.

Baron, M., Barkai, A., Gruen, R., Peselow, E., Fieve, R. R., & Quitkin, F. (1986). Platelet ^{3}H-imipramine binding in affective disorders: Trait versus state characteristics. *American Journal of Psychiatry, 143,* 711–717.

Bunney, W. E., Fawcett, J. A., Davis, J. M., & Gifford, S. (1969). Further evaluation of urinary 17-hydroxy-corticosteroid in suicidal patients. *Archives of General Psychiatry, 21,* 138–150.

Carroll, B. J. (1985). Dexamethasone suppression test: A review of contemporary confusion. *Journal of Clinical Psychiatry, 46,* 13–24.

Carroll, B. J., Feinberg, M., Greden, J. F., Tarika, J., Albala, A. A., Haskett, R. F., James N. M., Kronfol, Z., Lohr, N., Steiner, M., de Vigne, J. P., & Young, E. (1981). A specific laboratory test for the diagnosis of melancholia: Standardization, validation, and clinical utility. *Archives of General Psychiatry, 38,* 15–22.

Carroll, B. J., Greden, J. F., & Feinberg, M. (1981). Suicide, neuroendocrine dysfunction and CSF 5-HIAA concentrations in depression. In B. Angrist, G. D. Burrows, M. Lader (Eds.), *Recent advances in neuropsychopharmacology* (pp. 307–313). Elmsford, NY: Pergamon Press.

Davis, K. L., Davis, B. M., Mathea, A. A., Mohs, R. C., Rothpearl, A. B., Levy, M. I., Gorman, L. K., & Berger, P. (1984). Age and the dexamethasone suppression test in depression. *American Journal of Psychiatry, 141,* 872–874.

Georgotas, A., Schweitzer, J., McCue, R. E., Armour, M., & Friedhoff, A. J. (1987). Clinical and treatment effects on ³H-clonidine and ³H-imipramine binding in elderly depressed patients. *Life Sciences, 40,* 2137–2143.

Jones, J. S., Stanley, B., Mann, J. J., Frances, A. J., Guideo, J. R., Traskman-Bende, L., Winchel, R., Brown, R. P., & Stanley, M. (1990). CSF 5-HIAA and HVA concentrations in elderly depressed patients who attempted suicide. *American Journal of Psychiatry, 147,* 1225–1227.

Kellner, C. H., Rubinow, D. R., Gold, P. W., & Post, R. M. (1983). Relationship of cortisol hypersecretion to brain CT scan alterations in depressed patients. *Psychiatry Research, 8,* 191–197.

Kellner, C. H., Rubinow, D. R., & Post, R. M. (1986). Cerebral ventricular size and cognitive impairment in depression. *Journal of Affective Disorders, 10,* 215–219.

Langer, S. Z., Galzin, A. M., Poirier, M. F., Loo, H., Sechter, D., & Zarifian, E. (1987). Association of ³H-imipramine and ³H-paroxetine binding with the 5HT transporter in brain and platelets: Relevance to studies in depression. *Journal of Receptor Research, 7,* 499–521.

Langer, S. Z., Sechter, D., Loo, H., Raisman, R., & Zarifian, E. (1986). Electroconvulsive shock therapy and maximum binding of platelet tritiated imipramine binding in depression. *Archives of General Psychiatry, 43,* 949–952.

Lewis, D. A., & McChesney, C. (1985). Tritiated imipramine binding distinguishes among subtypes of depression. *Archives of General Psychiatry, 42,* 485–488.

Marcussen, J. O., Alafuzoff, I., Backstrom, I. T., Ericson, E., Gottfries, C. G., & Winblad, B. (1987). 5-hydroxytryptamine-sensitive 3H-imipramine binding of protein nature in the human brain. II. Effect of normal aging and dementia disorders. *Brain Research, 425,* 137–145.

Mellerup, E., & Langer, S. Z. (1990). Validity of imipramine platelet binding sites as a biological marker of endogenous depression. *Pharmacopsychiatry, 23,* 113–117.

Nemeroff, C. B., Knight, D. L., Krishnan, K. R. K., Slotkin, T. A., Bissette, G., Melville, M. L., & Blazer, D. G. (1988). Marked reduction in the number of platelet-tritiated ³H-imipramine binding sites in geriatric depression. *Archives of General Psychiatry, 45,* 919–923.

Nemeroff, C. B., Owens, M. J., Bissette, G., Andorn, A. C., & Stanley, M. (1988). Reduced corticotropin releasing factor binding sites in the frontal cortex of suicide victims. *Archives of General Psychiatry, 45,* 577–579.

Ostroff, R., Giller, E., Bonese, K., Ebersole, E., Harkness, L., & Mason, J. (1982). Neuroendocrine risk factors of suicidal behavior. *American Journal of Psychiatry, 139,* 1323–1325.

Owen, F., Chambers, D. R., Cooper, S. J., Crow, T. J., Johnson, J. A., Lofthouse, R., & Poulter, M. (1986). Serotonergic mechanisms in brains of suicide victims. *Brain Research, 362,* 185–188.

Rao, V. P., Krishnan, K. R., Goli, V., Saunders, W. B., Ellinwood, E. H., Blazer, D. G., & Nemeroff, C. B. (1989). Neuroanatomical changes and hypothalamo-pituitary-adrenal axis abnormalities. *Biological Psychiatry, 26,* 729–732.

Roy-Byrne, P., Post, R. M., Rubinow, D. R., Linnoila, M., Savard, R., & Davis, D. (1983). CSF 5-HIAA and personal and family history of suicide in affectively ill patients: A negative study. *Psychiatry Research, 10,* 263–274.

Schneider, L. S., Fredrickson, E., Severson, J., & Sloane, R. B. (1986). ^{3}H-imipramine binding in depressed elderly: Relationship to family history and clinical response. *Psychiatry Research, 19,* 257–266.

Schneider, L. S., Severson, J., Chui, H. C., Pollock, V. E., Sloane, R. B., & Fredrickson, E. R. (1988). ^{3}H-imipramine binding and MAO activity in Alzheimer's patients with agitation and delusions. *Psychiatry Research, 25,* 311–322.

Schneider, L. S., Severson, J. A., & Sloane, R. B. (1985). Platelet ^{3}H-imipramine binding in depressed elderly patients. *Biological Psychiatry, 20,* 1234–1237.

Schneider, L. S., Severson, J. A., Sloane, R. B., & Fredrickson, E. (1988). Decreased platelet ^{3}H-imipramine binding in primary major depression compared with depression secondary to medical illness in elderly outpatients. *Journal of Affective Disorders, 15,* 195–200.

Severson, J. A. (1986). ^{3}H-imipramine binding in aged mouse brain: Regulation by ions and serotonin. *Neurobiology of Aging, 7,* 83–87.

Severson, J. A., Marcussen, J. W., Osterburg, H. H., Finch, C. E., & Winblad, B. (1985). Elevated density of 3H-imipramine binding in aged human brain. *Journal of Neurochemistry, 45,* 1382–1389.

Stanley, M., & Mann, J. J. (1983). Serotonin-2 binding sites are increased in the frontal cortex of suicide victims. *Lancet, 1,* 214–216.

Stanley, M., Virgilio, J., & Gershon, S. (1982). Tritiated imipramine binding sites are decreased in frontal cortex of suicides. *Science, 216,* 1337.

Suranyi-Cadotte, B. E., Gauthier, S., Lafaille, F., Flores, S., Dam, T. V., Nair, N. P., & Quirion, R. (1985). Platelet ^{3}H-imipramine binding distinguishes depression from Alzheimer dementia. *Life Science, 37,* 2305–2311.

Targum, S. D., Rosen, L., & Capodanno, A. E. (1983). The dexamethasone suppression test in suicidal patients with unipolar depression. *American Journal of Psychiatry, 140,* 877–879.

Tourigny-Rivard, M. F., Raskind, M., & Rivard, D. (1981). The dexamethasone suppression test in an elderly population. *Biological Psychiatry, 16,* 1177–1184.

Wagner, A., Abert-Wistedt, A., Åsberg, M., Bertilsson, L., Martensson, B., & Montero, D. (1987). Effects of antidepressant treatments on platelet tritiated imipramine binding in major depressive disorder. *Archives of General Psychiatry, 44,* 870–877.

Weiner, M. F., Davis, B. M., Mohs, R. C., & Davis, K. L. (1987). Influence of age and relative weight on cortisol suppression in normal subjects. *American Journal of Psychiatry, 144,* 646–649.

Yerevanian, B., Olafsdottir, H., Milanese, E., Russotto, J., Mallon, P., Baciewicz, G., & Sagi, E. (1983). Normalization of the dexamethasone suppression test at discharge: Its prognostic value. *Journal of Affective Disorders, 5,* 191–197.

4

Suicide among Ethnic Elders

F. M. BAKER

The population of the United States is aging. The composition of the U.S. population is changing also. Ethnic minorities (African Americans, American Indians and Alaskan Natives, Asian Americans, and Hispanic Americans) will constitute the majority of the U.S. population within the next 30 years (Worobey & Hogan, 1991). The fastest growing segment of these populations are the "old-old" persons, aged 85 and older (National Center for Health Statistics, 1991). By the year 2030, 15.3% of persons age 65 and older will be members of these four groups. In 2050, ethnic elders will comprise 21.3% of the U.S. population (National Center for Health Statistics, 1991). Because numerically these groups will not be "minorities," the term ethnic elder is used; also, this term recognizes the unique place that these individuals usually hold in their families and cultures of origin.

There have been few studies of suicide among ethnic elders (McIntosh & Santos, 1985–1986; Seiden, 1981). Although focused on younger age cohorts, a few studies have reported on completed suicides across the life cycle (Baker, 1989; Hoppe & Martin, 1986; Miller, 1971; Yamamoto, 1976). Specific data on completed suicides for whites and blacks have been reported by the U.S. Census Bureau for decades. Enumeration of other ethnic populations has occurred only recently. Although data on American Indian and Alaskan Native populations are available from the Indian Health Service, there is little information on Asian American populations. Due to the increase in the U.S. Hispanic population, the U.S. Census Bureau changed its reporting format in 1980 to provide data on Hispanics (any race), Hispanics (white), and Hispanics (black). Although recent figures are available, longitudinal data are not available.

Attitudes toward suicide vary by ethnic group (Griffith et al., 1989a). Among the Japanese, the completion of a suicide is an acceptable, culturally sanctioned alternative to prevent embarrassment and to save face in interpersonal relationships. Other groups of ethnic elders consider suicide shameful (African Americans) or an act that has an adverse effect on the living (Navajo). After an overview of each group of ethnic elders, existing statistics on suicide will be presented. Where specific studies or existing literature are available, the attitude toward the completion of suicide by each group of ethnic elders will be discussed. The chapter will conclude with a summary of the known information and the areas where further investigation is indicated.

ETHNIC ELDERS: AN OVERVIEW

By the 1988 U.S. Census projections, African Americans make up 12% of the U.S. population, American Indians and Alaskan Natives make up 3% of the U.S. population, Asian Americans are 1% of the U.S. population, and Hispanic Americans are 8% of the total U.S. population (U.S. Bureau of the Census, 1988). Eleven percent of the African American population and 3% of the Hispanic American population are age 65 and older (Table 4–1). Six percent of Asian American and American Indian groups are age 65 and older (Table 4–1).

Describing the various groups of ethnic elders is a complex task because of the diversity within each group (Cuellar et al., 1982). Americans of African origin not only include African Americans whose families may have migrated from southern cities to the Midwest, Northeast, and West in the early 1900s but now refer to an increasing population of African Caribbeans who are recent immigrants to the United States (Baker, 1988). There are over 400 recognized American Indian and Alaskan Native tribes and over 250 languages (Manson & Callaway, 1988).

Asian Americans and Pacific Islanders denote two groups (Wykle & Kaskel, 1991). Asian Americans include persons who are Burmese, Cambodian, Chinese, East Indian, Indonesian, Japanese, Korean, Laotian, Malayan, Philippino, Thai, and Vietnamese. Pacific Islanders are Fijian, Guamian, Hawaiian, Micronesian, Samoan, and Tongan. Wykle and

TABLE 4–1

Ethnic Elders: Percentage of U.S. Population and Percentage of Ethnic Elders 65 and Over

Ethnic Elder Group (EEG)	Total U.S. Pop (%)	EEG Age 65+ (%)
African American	12	11
American Indian and Alaskan Native	1	6
Asian American	3	6
Hispanic American	8	3

Source: U.S. Bureau of the Census, 1990. National Center for Health Statistics. (1991). *Health: United States, 1990.* Hyattsville, MD: Public Health Service.

Kaskel note that each of these groups has its own history, religion, language, values, lifestyle, and pattern of immigration to the United States.

Hispanic elders, also, are a diverse grouping of persons with a common language and different genetic and cultural origins. In declining order of size, Mexican Americans, mainland Puerto Ricans, Cuban Americans, Central/South Americans, and other Latin backgrounds comprise this group (Baker, 1990).

The diversity and heterogeneity of these groups cannot be addressed within the narrow focus of this chapter. The reader is referred to a series of excellent monographs prepared by the Stanford Geriatric Education Center (Cuellar, 1990a, 1990b; Morioka-Douglas & Yeo, 1990; Richardson, 1990) and a Task Force Report of the American Psychiatric Association for detailed information about these groups (Sakauye et al., 1995). An additional excellent resource is a text edited by M. S. Harper (1990) that addressed essential curricular context for these populations of ethnic elders.

Problems with the U.S. Census data are acknowledged. Undercounting occurs because of inner-city vandalizing of mail boxes, individuals concerned about immigrant status who do not respond, and inaccurate addresses for families with marginal incomes, who move frequently. Additional confounds are the failure to enumerate Hispanic Americans separately until 1980. With 50% of American Indians resident in urban settings (John, 1991), available statistics on this population may not adequately reflect data on the nonreservation resident American Indian

TABLE 4–2
Education Attainment of Ethnic Elders, Aged 65–74

Ethnic Elder Group (EEG)	Completed College (%)	Completed High School (%)	Completed 5th and 6th Grade (%)	Without Any Formal Education (%)
African American	4	19	18	24
American Indian and Alaskan Native	4	25	11	23
Asian American	10	37	13	21
Hispanic American	4	20	18	35

Source: U.S. Bureau of the Census, 1990. National Center for Health Statistics. (1991). *Health: United States, 1990.* Hyattsville, MD: Public Health Service.

population. Further, the historically small population of Asian American and Pacific Islanders has recently increased, with the changing patterns of immigration. The complexity of this population has broadened.

Using the existing U.S. Census data, Table 4–2 presents educational attainment for ethnic elders aged 65–74, based on 1980 data. Asian American elders had the largest percentage of college graduates (10%) and American Indians and Alaskan Natives had the lowest percentage of persons who completed fifth and sixth grades (11%).

The percentage of individuals below the poverty level is presented in Table 4–3. African Americans had the largest percentage (35%) in

TABLE 4–3
Economic Status of Ethnic Elders: Percentage of Individuals and Households below the Poverty Level

Ethnic Elder Group (EEG)	Individuals below Poverty Level (%)	Households below Poverty Level (%)
African American	35	26
American Indian and Alaskan Native	25	—
Rural residents	39	
Asian American	14	—
Rural residents	10	
Hispanic American	26	21

Source: U.S. Bureau of the Census, 1990.

contrast to Asian Americans with only 14% of individuals below the poverty level. Data on households below the poverty level were available for only African Americans and Hispanic Americans. American Indians and Alaskan Natives had the largest percentage (39%) of persons who were rural residents, a factor that is closely linked with poverty (Cuellar, 1990a).

African Americans

The African American and African Caribbean populations are the majority African origin populations in the United States. The recent increased immigration of African Caribbeans will result in a greater emphasis on language and acculturation in black elders in 2020. The current cohort of black elders are predominantly African American and are 12% of the total U.S. population. Persons age 65 and older are 11% of the total African American population.

Born in the southern United States in the early 1900s, these elders learned from their grandparents and their great-grandparents of their African heritage, a value system that emphasized family, community concerns above individual concerns, collectivity, affiliation, and the role of the elder in providing wisdom and leadership (Baker, 1987). African American elders learned of their African heritage from oral historians. Although chattel slavery intentionally mixed individuals from different tribal groups who spoke different languages, continuity of history was maintained. The historical life event calendar for the African American elder has been described in a few contexts (Baker, 1982; Baker & Lightfoot, 1995). Briefly, such elders grew up in the South, migrated to metropolitan centers in the early 1900s, and may look forward to returning to their birthplace during retirement (Longino & Smith, 1991). Having lived through three wars, three police actions, and two black liberation movements (the "Back to Africa" movement of Marcus Garvey and the Black Revolution of the 1960s), these African American elders have seen the ending of segregation, the expansion of opportunities for their children and grandchildren, and the economic and political retrenchment that began in the 1980s.

These African American elders experienced inadequate medical and psychiatric resources for the majority of their lives because of segregated health care services (Prudhomme & Musto, 1973). Depending on alternative health care systems, they consulted root doctors and used "natural medicines" (teas from roots and plants) to manage their medical problems

(Richardson, 1990). Although Medicare has provided an improved economic base for care and community mental health centers are located within their communities, African American elders continue to be under-utilizers of health care resources. The increased prevalence of chronic diseases (diabetes, arthritis [primarily osteoarthritis], hypertension, heart disease, asthma, glaucoma, gout, and goiter) place them at increased risk for major depressive disorders (Baker, Lavisso-Mourey, & Jones, in press).

Due to the loss of African American males aged 20 to 35 because of mortality from homicide, suicide, and accidents, the gender ratio is reduced by the fourth decade of life. Between the ages 65 and 74, there are 67 men per 100 women. For the age group 85 and older, there are 46 men per 100 women.

Few studies have assessed the presence of psychopathology in older African Americans. In one study in which 40% of the sample from an ambulatory family practice setting was African American, one third of these patients were diagnosed as being depressed and 31% screened positive for depressive symptoms (Rosenthal, Goldfarb, Carlson, Sagi, & Balaban, 1987).

American Indians and Alaskan Natives

This U.S. Census category includes American Indians and Alaskan Natives (Eskimos and Aleuts). These are over 400 distinct tribal groups with over 250 different languages besides English. As noted by Cuellar (1990a), the designation Native American reflects, also, a particular political relationship to both federal and state governments that involves specific political rights and benefits to citizens whose descent includes at least one-fourth "Indian blood." Several authors have emphasized the increased "functional dependence" of American Indian elders at a younger chronological age because of the earlier onset of "old age" problems. Manson and Callaway (1988) have documented that an American Indian aged 55 addresses medical and psychosocial problems similar to a white American aged 65. The long history of inequity of services, treaty negotiations, and genocidal acts are detailed in other sources (Block, 1979; Brown, 1971; Clevenger, 1982). The long marches to resettlement on reservations, frequently very different from their initial lands, and the provision of small-pox-infested blankets are two examples, widely known, of detrimental acts involving American Indian populations.

Less than 1% of the total U.S. population, persons age 65 and older, represent 6% of the American Indian and Alaskan Native population (U.S. Bureau of the Census, 1988). Nationally, 54% of American Indians live in predominantly urban areas with less than 24% living on reservations (John, 1991). The gender ratio is significantly reduced. In the group aged 65 to 74, there are 77 men per 100 women; and for age 85 and older, there are 59 men per 100 women.

The major health problems of American Indians and Alaskan Natives include non-insulin-dependent diabetes mellitus, hypertension, tuberculosis, heart disease, cancer, liver, and kidney disease. Psychiatric disorders include alcohol abuse with significant intertribal variation and alcohol dependence. Manson, Walker, and Kivlahan (1987) have assessed the use of the CES-D to screen older American Indian populations for depressive illness and found the instrument useful. An estimation of depressive disorder ranging from 30% to 50% has been made based on the evaluation of five tribal groups in the southwestern United States.

ASIAN AMERICANS AND PACIFIC ISLANDERS

This category of ethnic elders includes individuals with more than 20 different ethnicities with origins in East Asia, Southeast Asia, the Indian subcontinent, Polynesia, Melanesia, and Micronesia. Representing 1% of the total U.S. population, 6% of the Asian/Pacific Islander population is age 65 and older. Sixty-four percent of these ethnic elders live in California, Hawaii, and Washington in declining order of residence, with 90% living in urban areas. Sixty-five percent were born outside the United States. The three largest groups are Chinese, Japanese, and Filipino (Morioko-Douglas & Yeo, 1990).

A biphasic immigration pattern resulted from discriminatory legislation. In the late 1800s to early 1900s, often unmarried and poorly educated male immigrants from China, Japan, and the Philippines immigrated to the United States to provide cheap manual labor. Intending to make their fortunes before returning home or bringing their families to the United States, these plans did not materialize (Baker, 1990). Legislation halted immigration and naturalization of Asian groups beginning with the Chinese Exclusion Act of 1882 and ending with the Immigration Act of 1924, which barred the entry of all Asian populations. Legal sanctions against intermarriage and informal sanctions resulted in these early, predominantly male, immigrants becoming a "bachelor society." The repeal of these Asian Exclusion Acts in 1965 resulted in a second wave of immigration that included more Asian women, the older wives who had been excluded (Morioka-Douglas & Yeo, 1990).

Morioka-Douglas and Yeo (1990) note that of foreign-born Asian Americans and Pacific Islanders aged 65 and older in 1990, 86% were Japanese, 52% Filipino, 47% Asian Indians, and 37% Chinese. Salcido, Nakano, and Jue (1980) reported that of the 100 low-income Asian subjects aged 55 and older in Asian ethnic communities in Los Angeles, 75% spoke only their native language with 77% stating that they had resided in the United States for over 20 years.

Morbidity and mortality data are very different for these elders. Death rates were lower for Chinese, Japanese, and Filipinos (the only statistics on the various Asian/Pacific Islander groups that were kept by the National Center on Health Statistics) compared with the rate for whites.

Specific population-based studies have found lower rates of mortality due to coronary artery disease and acute myocardial infarction and a higher incidence of liver and esophageal cancers as well as multi-infarct dementia in Chinese populations (Morioka-Douglas & Yeo, 1990). Second-generation (Nisei) Japanese Americans were found to have 3 to 6 times the rate of non-insulin-dependent diabetes mellitus as white U.S. males, to lack higher kidney-related complications among diabetics, to have a higher incidence of stomach cancer in Japanese living in the United States, and to have higher suicide rates for Japanese women 75 years and older and Issei (first-generation) Japanese age 85 and older (Morioka-Douglas & Yeo, 1990).

HISPANIC AMERICANS

Cuellar (1990b) notes that the term "Hispanic" is an overarching term that bridges pertinent national, ethnic, and racial variations in a heterogeneous population. He emphasizes that Hispanic Americans range from native-born U.S. citizens to documented political-economic refugees from certain Latin American socialist governments (i.e., Cubans and Nicaraguans). The earliest immigrants to the continental United States were from Mexico and Puerto Rico. They were followed by Cuban immigrants who fled the Castro Revolution followed by Salvadorians, Nicaraguans, and Colombians (Baker, 1990). Although 8% of the total

U.S. population, the Hispanic American population is a younger population. Its young median age, high fertility rates, and immigration status combine to result in a pattern of escalating population growth (Cuellar, 1990b). Of the three largest groups of Hispanic Americans, the percentage of persons age 65 and older varies; for the Cuban population 11.7%, for Mexican Americans 4.2%, for Puerto Ricans 3.6%, and for Central/South Americans 2.8%. The gender ratio is distinct. For U.S. Hispanics aged 60–64, there are 86 men for every 100 women. At age 85, there are 61 men for every 100 women. Although the majority of Hispanic Americans have higher mortality rates, which have been related to the "stress, wear, and tear" of birthing and raising large numbers of children, mortality and morbidity data are lacking in general because large-scale studies have not been done (Cuellar, 1990b). For the most part, existing studies are case reports, Lacuyo (1980) reported that arthritis, hypertension, circulation problems, and diabetes mellitus were the primary diseases of concern. Intergroup differences are suggested by existing data. Mexican-born persons had a rate of death due to accidents that was twice that of Puerto Rican born and Cuban-born populations. Mexican-born persons had the highest cerebrovascular disease mortality rates and Cuban-born persons the lowest. The mortality rates of Puerto Ricans due to chronic liver disease and cirrhosis were twice those of Mexicans and three times those of Cubans. Mortality rates due to homicide were high in all groups, but highest among Puerto Ricans. Suicide was highest among Cuban and Puerto Rican males and lowest among females, particularly Mexican females (Cuellar, 1990b).

Only a few studies have looked at psychiatric disorders in older persons. Kemp, Staples, and Lopez-Aqueres (1987) used a regrouped set of Comprehensive Assessment and Referral Evaluation (CARE) items in an area-probability sampling of 700 older Hispanics living in Los Angeles County to reflect criteria of the *Diagnostic and Statistical Manual of Mental Disorders* (DSM-III-R; American Psychiatric Association, 1987). These authors found more than 26% of the population with depression or dysphoria. Affective disorder was found to correlate strongly with medical disability and, also, with dementia.

Issues of exclusion based on ethnicity, level of acculturation, and language vary for each component of the Hispanic American population. Mexican Americans who have a unique history in the development of the southwestern United States represent a population ranging from initial landowners and indigenous residents, who were displaced with

the Mexican War and the formation of the state of Texas, to the undocu-
mented worker of the 1990s who moves fluidly between Mexico and the
United States, but who suffers the chronic psychosocial stresses of con-
stant vigilance for immigration authorities as well as exploitation by em-
ploying farmers (Martinez, 1988).

DATA ON SUICIDE AMONG ETHNIC ELDERS

According to the 1988 U.S. Census data (Table 4–4), Asian American elders had the highest rates of completed suicide (11.5 per 100,000 population) and African American elders had the lowest rate of 6.6 per 100,000
population. When the probability of lifetime suicide was compared by
race and gender (data available for only a black-white comparison), the
calculated relative risks were highest for men and lowest for women
(Table 4–5). The relative risk of the probability of lifetime suicide by
black men was one half the relative risk of white men and for black
women was almost one third the risk of white women. Specific rates of
completed suicide by American Indians and Alaskan Natives were obtained from data provided by the Indian Health Service (Table 4–6). The
rates among American Indian elders are the lowest for the four groups of
ethnic elders. An interesting pattern of a decline in the group aged 75 to
84 to one half the rate observed in the group aged 65 to 74 followed by a
return in the 85+ age group to a rate similar to the group aged 65 to 74 requires further evaluation.

Only for African American elders are longitudinal data available because of the historic enumeration of white-black data by the U.S. Census

TABLE 4–4
Completed Suicides by Ethnic Elders, Aged 65 and Over (1988 Data)

Race	Number of Deaths	Rate per 100,000	SE (Rate)
White	6,139	22.5	(0.3)
Black	164	6.6	(0.5)
American Indian/ Alaskan Native	7	6.7	(2.5)
Asian	53	11.5	(1.6)
Hispanic (any race)	74	10.3	(1.2)

Source: National Center for Health Statistics. Unpublished data (1988), U.S.
Public Health Service, Hyattsville, MD.

TABLE 4–5
Probability of Lifetime Suicide—Race and Gender Comparisons

	Probability	*Relative Risk*
Black Female	1 out of 535	1.0
White Female	1 out of 196	2.7
Black Male	1 out of 133	4.0
White Male	1 out of 66	8.1

Source: U.S. Decennial Life Table for 1979–1981, Vol. 1, No. 2, National Center for Health Statistics, 1988, U.S. Public Health Service, Hyattsville, MD.

Bureau. Table 4–7 provides an overview of the last 8 years of completed suicides per 100,000 population by age group, race, and gender based on data from *Health United States, 1990* (National Center for Health Statistics, 1991). The data do not document a reported pattern of an increase in completed suicide by African American men age 85 and older (Griffith & Bell, 1989).

CROSS-CULTURAL ATTITUDES TOWARD SUICIDE

One of the most comprehensive reviews of suicide among these four ethnic groups is the monograph prepared by the Committee on Cultural Psychiatry of the Group for the Advancement of Psychiatry (GAP). This

TABLE 4–6
Comparison of Total American Indian and Alaskan Native Suicide Death Rates to the Total U.S. Population All Races and U.S. Population (other than white) Suicide Death Rates

Age Group	*American Indian and Alaskan Native*	*U.S. All Races*	*U.S. Other than White*
65–74	9.3 M = 14.7 F = 4.8	19.7 M = 35.5 F = 7.2	9.2 M = 6.9 F = 3.5
74–84	3.1 M = 7.1 F = —	25.2 M = 54.8 F = 7.5	8.3 M = 16.4 F = 3.1
85+	5.5 M = 13.7 F = —	20.8 M = 61.6 F = 4.7	7.8 M = 20.0 F = 1.8

Source: U.S. Bureau of Indian Affairs. *American Indian Health.* (1990). Washington, DC: U.S. Department of Health and Human Services.

TABLE 4–7
Suicide Death Rates by Age, Race, and Gender in the United States—Selected Years

	1980	*1984*	*1986*	*1988*
65–74				
All races	16.9	18.8	19.7	18.4
White males	32.5	35.6	37.6	35.4
White females	7.0	7.8	7.7	7.3
Black males	11.1	13.8	16.1	12.9
Black females	1.7	2.5	2.8	2.0
75–84				
All races	19.1	22.0	25.2	25.9
White males	45.5	52.0	58.9	61.5
White females	5.7	6.8	8.0	7.4
Black males	10.5	15.1	16.0	17.6
Black females	1.4	0.5	2.6	1.3
85 Years and Over				
All races	19.2	18.4	20.8	20.5
White males	52.8	55.8	66.3	65.8
White females	5.8	5.1	5.0	5.3
Black males	18.9	11.1	17.9	10.0
Black females	—	0.8	—	—

Source: National Center for Health Statistics. *Health. United States, 1990,* U.S. Public Health Service, Hyattsville, MD.

monograph entitled *Group for the Advancement of Psychiatry: Report No. 128. Suicide and Ethnicity in the United States* (Griffith et al., 1989a) provides an extensive analysis of cultural, attitudinal, societal, and psychosocial factors contributing to a specific ethnic group's attitude toward suicide.

African Americans

The rate of completed suicide declines with age. Although two studies noted an increase in completed suicide between 1970 and 1985 in African American men aged 85 and older (Baker, 1989; Griffith & Bell, 1989), data from 1980 to 1988 did not confirm an ongoing trend. The rates of completed suicide by black women remained consistently low (Baker, 1989). Various authors attempted to provide explanations for this gender difference. Hendin (1969) suggested that a family history of childhood violence resulted in an intense struggle to deal with unconscious rage and murderous impulses, particularly for black males. Bush (1976) suggested that intragroup pressure ("the black perspective") or the collective experience common to black Americans, could be a buffer or a negative force for suicide. This author suggested that an African American rejecting the black perspective and experiencing the African American perspective as a negative value orientation would become a "depreciated character" who might seek suicide as a solution to his dilemma (Bush, 1976). As summarized in the GAP report, "intragroup solidarity decreased the black individual's risk of experiencing identity confusion" (Griffith et al., 1989b). King (1982) emphasized the sociopolitical context of blacks in the United States. Daily confronting racism, oppression, and violent treatment from whites, power (defined as the feeling, real or imagined, that one could create a change) was a key variable. Without this feeling, an individual would respond with a malignant sense of helplessness that could lead to suicide, depending on the degree at which the individual felt empowered or powerless. These explanations do not address the lower rates for black females. Baker (1989) suggested that the extended family and the important role of the church (Comer, 1973) provided alternative settings that reinforced the African American female's self-esteem. Wylie (1971) emphasized the importance of alternative roles for older African Americans when the role of work was ended with retirement. The roles of elder in the family, grandparent, community leader, and elder in the church were all available to the African American elder in retirement, which resulted in enhanced self-esteem, mastery, and a sense of productivity. The significantly lower suicide rates among African Americans in the South are related to the strength of the black church and black family in the rural South (Griffith, et al., 1989b).

Henry and Short (1954) presented an alternative model for explaining the presence or absence of suicide. Their external restraint theory suggested that suicide varied inversely with horizontal restraining factors (social relationships with others) and vertical restraining factors (social class and/or social status). These authors and Maris (1969) defined the strength of the relational system of the individual by marital status, urban-rural residence, and ecological distribution. The stronger the relational system, the lower the number of suicides. Davis (1980) questioned whether a decrease in overt racism and discrimination, which fostered group solidarity, would decrease the relational system for African Americans. If this did occur, family ties would be left as the major insulation against the daily psychosocial stressors. Disorganized, overstressed, and/or dysfunctional families would be unable to provide ameliorating or buffering factors. In this context, the African American would be at higher risk for suicidal behavior. The African American elder with children resident at a distance and with siblings and friends deceased could have increased vulnerability to complete a suicide based on this conceptual model.

Suicide is not culturally sanctioned in African American culture. Such an act brings shame to the person and his or her family. The GAP report notes (Griffith et al., 1989b) that blacks in the South have lower socioeconomic expectations and may be less at risk to becoming enraged with their life circumstances. An alternative explanation of marginality as a conceptual model resulting in suicides was presented (Griffith et al., 1989b). Here, the African American individual rejects his or her identity and rejects positive relations with whites. By rejecting both cultural contexts, the individual is left without ties to either community. This conceptual model was used to explain the increased rates of suicide among African American males age 85 and over. It was suggested that these elders withdrew voluntarily into the segregated black community after following a pattern of integrative adaptation (positive self-identity and positive relations with whites). Further study of these hypotheses was encouraged by the Committee on Cultural Psychiatry (Griffith et al., 1989b). The GAP Committee questioned whether as blacks achieved more financial success, they might experience the retirement years as being more unpleasant and more of a sociopsychological letdown (Griffith et al., 1989b).

In her review of completed suicide by African Americans, Baker (1989) addressed specific preventive strategies. Primary preventive strategies included the removal of outdated medications from the home to decrease the availability of medications to the distraught individual making an impulsive act. Further, the importance of prescribing non-lethal amounts of medication to persons in active treatment for psychiatric disorders was underscored. Secondary preventive strategies emphasized the importance of including the person accompanying the suicide attempter in the psychiatric assessment. A crisis intervention at the time of the initial evaluation would facilitate conflict resolution and, possibly, improve compliance with the referral to outpatient treatment. The use of involuntary hospitalization must be considered for the persistently suicidal person who does not follow through on referrals to treatment. Tertiary preventive strategies focus on the surviving significant others of the person who has completed a suicide. This postventive work is important in facilitating the clarification of feelings, acknowledging and addressing the anger and ambivalence of the survivors, and providing a structured setting to facilitate this complex grieving process.

American Indians and Alaskan Natives

The complexity of American Indian and Alaskan Native populations preclude any generalizations about the attitude of the various recognized tribal groups toward suicide. The perspective of the Navajo, one of the largest tribal groups, is presented (Griffith et al., 1989c). The Navajo people emphasize a religious-philosophical perspective that emphasizes living in harmony with nature. This pattern of harmony can be disrupted by a witch who casts a spell on the individual. A Navajo person who completes a suicide is believed to have been influenced by a witch. The Navajo people do not emphasize the loss of the person who completes the suicide, but focus on the harm this action inflicts on the living. The dead person will continue to wander as a ghost, placing the living at risk. For the Navajo, suicide does not resolve an intolerable situation, it causes the victim to remain in the situation as a ghost (Griffith et al., 1989c).

American Indians having more contact with the dominant society (one measure of acculturation) were found to have higher suicide rates (Van Winkle & May, 1986). Navajos, in contrast to other tribes (e.g., Apache and Uto-Aztecian), have continued to emphasize the uniqueness of their culture and crafts and have minimized contacts with the dominant culture (Van Winkle & May, 1986). Where traditional roles such as spiritual leader, priest, and minister have been usurped by white religious leaders, loss of role definition was believed to contribute to the pattern of observed suicide (Griffith et al., 1989c). For a discussion of completed suicide in Southwest Indians, Pueblo Indians, Pacific Northwest Indians, Intermountain Indians, Northern Plains Indians, Boreal Forest Indians, and Arctic Indians, the reader is referred to the GAP monograph (Griffith et al., 1989c) and the National Center for American Indians and Alaskan Natives Mental Health Research at the University of Colorado Health Science Center (303-270-4600).

Asian Americans and Pacific Islanders

Intragroup variance in attitudes toward suicide are strikingly exemplified by the difference between Japanese and Chinese cultural attitudes toward suicide. Japanese culture has sanctioned ritual suicide for the samurai warrior class, termed *seppuku,* as an appropriate method for handling failure or atoning for an inappropriate act. An example (Griffith et al., 1989d) is the story of the 47 samurai who tracked down and killed those persons responsible for the death of their master. Then, all 47 samurai committed ritual suicide, seppuku (also called hara-kiri), to atone for the murders they had committed. Japanese civilians may complete suicide as a resolution to a difficult situation or to atone for losing face. The story of the Lady Tekona (Griffith et al., 1989d) illustrates this. Not wishing to embarrass either of two ardent suitors, she resolved her interpersonal relationship dilemma by completing a suicide. With her suicide, her suitors completed suicide, also. A Shinto temple memorializes this woman who, even to this day, is honored as one who exemplifies the importance of saving face in interpersonal relationships (Griffith et al., 1989d). Japanese men who are depressed by the material competitiveness of their economy frequently select suicide as a way to opt out of the "rat race," as described by Matsugi (1980). Comparative studies of suicide between Japan, China, and Taiwan are shown in Table 4–8. The rates of suicide are highest for Japanese in Japan.

In Chinese culture, there is no sanction of suicide. Cultural belief systems were influenced by the teachings of Confucius, which emphasized harmony in the home, propriety between husband and wife, and a traditional, sexist, hierarchical society (Griffith et al., 1989d). Living a good life guided by these principles is emphasized. The rates of suicide among Chinese Americans are lower in comparison with that of white Americans

TABLE 4–8

Comparison of Completed Suicide in Japan and by Chinese in Hong Kong and Chinese in Taiwan (1977–1980)

Country	Rates of Suicide per 100,000 Population
Japanese in Japan	17.8
Chinese in Taiwan	9.8
Japanese in Japan	23.4
Chinese in Hong Kong	14.2

Note: Data from "Suicide among the Chinese and the Japanese," by E. E. H. Griffith, A. K. Delgado, E. Foulks, et al. (1989), in *Group for the Advancement of Psychiatry: Report No. 128. Suicide and ethnicity in the United States* (pp. 42–43). New York: Brunner/Mazel. Copyright 1989 by Brunner/Mazel. Used by permission.

(see Table 4–9). Unlike the majority of other groups, Chinese American and Japanese American women have increasing rates of suicide after age 55; rates which increase with increasing age. At age 85 and older, the rate for Chinese American women is 49.9 per 100,000 in contrast to a rate of 4.9 for white women. The role of cohort experience and marginality are presented as explanations of the observed data (Griffith et al., 1989d). The repeal of the Oriental Exclusion Acts in 1965 was the first opportunity for a number of Chinese women to enter the United States. Many older women possessed few marketable skills. They experienced cultural tension between traditional Chinese values emphasizing family and the central role of women and American culture emphasizing equality of the sexes. These older women experience poverty without the support of the traditional family (Griffith et al., 1989d). These factors are identified as contributing to the high rates of suicide observed among elderly Chinese women. A similar explanation of the high suicide rate among Japanese women is suggested with specific emphasis on isolation due to the loss of family members.

Older Chinese men are a "bachelor cohort." Immigrating before 1924, the Oriental Exclusion Act of 1924 prevented them from bringing

TABLE 4–9
U.S. Average Annual Age-Specific and Age-Adjusted Suicide Rates per 100,000 Population for Specified Races 1980—Age 55 to Age 85

Age Group	Chinese			Japanese			White		
	Total	Male	Female	Total	Male	Female	Total	Male	Female
All ages, crude	8.27	8.26	8.28	9.08	12.57	6.14	13.31	20.57	6.43
Age adjusted	7.97	7.93	8.02	7.84	11.08	5.00	12.54	19.41	6.20
55–64 years	12.34	9.37	15.52	9.93	12.38	7.78	17.54	26.52	9.59
65–74 years	24.35	25.85	22.61	6.61	11.17	2.17	18.28	32.41	7.45
75–84 years	33.51	21.82	44.32	25.01	39.56	15.75	20.91	46.18	6.03
85+ years	56.13	64.10	49.93	62.59	139.76	19.50	19.45	53.28	4.92

Source: W. Liu & E. Yu, Division of Vital Statistics, National Center for Health Statistics. Unpublished data, 1985, U.S. Public Health Service, Hyattsville, MD.

their families to the United States. They are alone, have marginal resources, experience acculturation stress without the traditional cultural context, and have not established a positive relationship with the dominant culture. They are at an increased risk to complete a suicide and have higher suicide rates.

Hispanic Americans

Although a significant proportion of Hispanic groups are Catholic, the strong religious condemnation of suicide has not resulted in uniformly low rates of completed suicide in Mexican American, Puerto Rican, and Cuban groups. In one of the few triracial studies of suicide completed by Monk and Warshauer (1974) in New York City in 1968–1974, the highest rates of suicide were observed among Puerto Rican men age 18 and over with rates of 44.5 per 100,000 (Table 4–10). Rates reported for white men were 31.5 per 100,000 and 29.6 per 100,000 for black men. Again, issues of acculturation are discussed (Smith, Mercy, & Warren, 1985) as contributing to these statistics. Referring to Durkheim's original conceptualization of anomie (Durkheim, 1951), these authors suggested that Puerto Rican immigrants experienced significant adjustment issues moving from rural Puerto Rico where the Anglo influence could be ignored to the mainland with its cultural pluralism and different value system. In a study of 67 Puerto Ricans living in a low-income neighborhood in Hartford, Connecticut, Dressler and Bernal (1982) found "the worst stress outcomes occurred in those persons who had been in the Anglo cultural environment the longest, but who did not have the resources for coping with that environment." These authors found that the availability of

TABLE 4–10

Annual Age-Adjusted Rate per 100,000 and Median Age for Persons Aged 18 and Over Who Completed Suicide in the East Harlem Section of New York City by Ethnic Group and Age, 1968–1970

	White		Puerto Rican		Black	
	Male	*Female*	*Male*	*Female*	*Male*	*Female*
Rate	31.5	32.5	44.5	17.5	29.6	10.7
Number	17	22	20	10	28	9
Median Age	50	40	27	30	35	40

Note: Data from "Completed and Attempted Suicide in Three Ethnic Groups," by M. Monk, & M. E. Warshauer, 1974, *American Journal of Epidemiology 100*(4), 333–345.

psychosocial resources from their own (Puerto Rican) culture or the dominant culture had a significant influence on altering the length of residence in the area and the number of (presumed) stress-related health problems. Being able to identify some commonality between these two disparate cultural contexts was the task. Individuals who were unable to resolve the discongruence in experiences, felt isolated from their culture of origin, and rejected the new mainland city culture were at increased risk to complete a suicide.

The pattern of suicide of Mexican Americans is different (Griffith et al., 1989e). Rates are reported as lower, but national data do not exist. Smith et al. (1985) studied 36,000 completed suicides in 5 states (Arizona, California, Colorado, New Mexico, and Texas). Table 4–11 shows the reported rates. From age 50, the rates of suicide for Mexican Americans increased, but were ½ to ⅓ the rates of Non-Hispanics in the five states. The rates of Mexican American women were low (the highest rate of 6.2 per 100,000 was found in the 40–49 age group) and declined throughout the life cycle. In contrast, the rates of completed suicide were

TABLE 4–11
Rates of Completed Suicide per 100,000 Persons in Five Southwestern States,*
1976–1980

Age	Total	Non-Hispanic Male	Female	Total	Hispanic Male	Female
0–15	0.5	0.7	0.2	0.2	0.3	0.1
15–19	11.9	18.6	5.2	9.0	14.8	3.4
20–24	23.3	37.4	9.7	18.7	33.1	5.4
25–29	24.6	36.4	12.2	16.0	26.4	6.1
30–39	22.6	30.7	14.4	14.7	23.8	6.2
40–49	24.8	31.0	18.6	12.2	18.2	6.5
50–59	26.4	34.4	18.9	11.8	19.8	4.7
60–69	26.7	40.9	14.8	11.7	20.0	4.4
70+	32.8	63.2	13.7	14.2	28.0	3.0
Total	19.2	27.5	11.2	9.0	14.6	3.5
Age-Adjusted Total	18.5	27.6	10.6	10.5	17.8	4.0

*Arizona, California, Colorado, New Mexico, and Texas.

Note: Data from "Hispanic suicide: Report for five southwestern states for the years 1976–1980," by J. C. Smith, J. A. Mercy, & C. W. Warren, 1985, *Suicide and Life-Threatening Behavior, 1*(1), 14–26. Copyright 1985 by Human Sciences Press, NY. Used by permission.

significantly lower in Mexican American women resident in Mexico (the highest rate of 0.8 per 100,000 was found in the 35–44 age group in 1973; see Table 4–12).

The GAP Committee (Griffith et al., 1989f) suggested that the erosion of the extended family caused by the influence of American culture resulted in a change in role for the older Mexican American men, the traditional patriarch. When children leave home earlier, move away, and live farther away, there is less sense of family and a decreased sense of family support. As a result, the anticipated respected role of grandparent may not occur and the Mexican American man will experience role loss, decreased self-esteem, and marginality. Factors identified as protecting the Mexican American woman from suicide are the intact nuclear family unit enabling the Mexican American woman to remain within her traditional role whether employed only within the home or outside the home as well.

In summary, peak rates of suicide among Mexican Americans occur in young adults and older men. Burnam et al. (1987) found that a group of Mexican Americans who were "more acculturated" had increased lifetime rates of phobia, alcohol abuse, and drug abuse or dependence. A higher prevalence of major depression and dysthymic disorder in Mexican Americans compared with persons born in Mexico was also observed. The authors explained their findings as related to the increased

TABLE 4–12
Suicide Rates in Mexico per 100,000 Population

Age	1965			1970			1973		
	Total	Males	Females	Total	Males	Females	Total	Males	Females
1–4	—	—	—	—	—	—	—	—	—
5–14	0.2	0.2	0.1	—	—	—	—	—	—
15–24	2.9	3.4	2.5	1.9	2.9	1.0	1.3	1.9	0.7
25–34	2.8	4.1	1.5	2.0	3.3	0.8	1.2	1.8	0.5
35–44	2.9	5.0	0.9	2.2	3.7	0.8	1.2	2.2	0.8
45–54	3.0	5.4	0.9	1.8	3.2	0.4	1.2	1.9	0.4
55–64	2.8	4.5	1.1	3.0	5.0	0.9	1.4	2.5	0.3
65–74	4.7	8.0	1.6	2.4	4.6	0.3	1.7	3.3	0.1
75+	7.0	8.4	5.6	3.7	7.7	0.3	1.6	2.9	0.5
All ages	1.7	2.4	1.0	1.1	1.8	0.5	0.7	1.1	0.3

Source: World Health Organization (1965, 1970, 1973). *World Health Statistics Annual.* Geneva.

stress associated with the "frustration of status expectations." Factors potentially contributing to a higher incidence of depressive spectrum illness among Mexican Americans are language barriers, cultural barriers, and forced family separation, potentially resulting in an affective illness and suicide.

RESEARCH CONCERNS

Suicide among older African American, American Indian and Alaskan Native, Asian American and Pacific Islander, and Hispanic American populations is a complex issue (Griffith et al., 1989f). In addition to the heterogeneity of the cultural context for each group, Warshauer and Monk (1978) presented specific data on how suicide statistics were flawed. In their New York City sample, African Americans who completed a suicide used "unusual" methods (jumping from tall buildings), did not have a request for a final determination of death made, and a change in the coding for the International Classification of Diseases resulted in these deaths being classified as assigned suicides. As only definite suicides were reported to the National Center for Health Statistics, these authors identified how statistics on completed suicides by African Americans in New York City in 1973 could have been underreported locally and nationally. The extent to which this is a concern for all groups of ethnic elders requires further study. These authors raise the important issue of the validity of the data that are used to plan services.

The rates of completed suicide for elderly ethnic groups are lower than for group members aged 15 to 44, where the rates of homicide (for all groups except Asian Americans) and suicide are highest. Deaths due to motor vehicle accidents are highest for American Indians. Although the rates are generally lower for these ethnic elders compared with older whites, there are critical exceptions. Older Chinese men, a cohort who were isolated from their families by the Oriental Exclusion Act of 1924, have the highest rates of completed suicide for the old-old, but are lower than for older Japanese Americans, where suicide is culturally sanctioned. Another exception is the increased rates of suicide observed in older Chinese American and Japanese American women, rates that increase with increasing age and are related to loss of traditional roles with death of spouse, loss of siblings, and separation from children. The rates of completed suicide by Hispanic subgroups vary depending on the level of acculturation and the individual's resolution of his or her bicultural or tricultural heritage. National data on Hispanic populations are only now beginning to be collected. Rates of completed suicide are lowest among older African American men and women probably reflecting the number of continuing roles after retirement and the support of the extended kinship network.

It is important to note that the data previously presented are specific for ethnic elders aged 65 to 85 years old in 1992 (born between 1907 and 1927). Legalized segregation, the Oriental Exclusion Acts, disputes over Indian territory/tribal lands and resettlement, and immigration status are part of the history of these ethnic elders. Ethnic elders who will reach ages 65 to 85 years old in 2050 were born between 1965 and 1985. These birth cohorts experienced the Civil Rights movement of the 1950s, the Black Revolution of the 1960s, a presidential assassination, Watergate, two presidential assassination attempts, the Iran-Contra hearings, and the savings and loan scandal, with more historical events to come. These ethnic elders of 2050 will be better educated, will have had a broader range of opportunities for employment, and should have had a decline in cardiovascular disease, hypertension, obesity, and diabetes with the adoption of a healthier lifestyle and diet. The types of psychosocial stressors as well as psychosocial resources, such as the extended family, may not exist in the same way for this cohort of ethnic elders (Markides & Mindel, 1987). Adult children may have moved several hundred miles away for better employment opportunities and these ethnic elders may have chosen to live in integrated suburban communities instead of homogenous ethnic enclaves.

Much needs to be studied to fully understand the etiology and psychological context for ethnic elder suicide (Carter, 1988; Fellin & Powell, 1988; Hoppe & Martin, 1986; Liu & Yu, 1985; Mercer, 1989; Pine, 1981; Westermeyer, 1979). Although there is suggestive evidence that because of associated multiple, chronic medical problems, African American, American Indian and Alaskan Native, and Hispanic American elders may be at increased risk to develop a depressive illness, specific studies of the incidence and prevalence of depression, dementia, and psychosis have not been done (Baker, 1991; Escobar et al., 1986; Manson, Shore, & Bloom, 1985; Markides, 1986). As suicide is a behavior and not a psychiatric diagnosis, it will be important, also, to understand the psychopathology underlying the suicidal act. Research in several phases is required to detect the problem across groups, to identify specific psychological contexts contributing to suicide, and to establish the specific psychiatric diagnoses associated with suicide in ethnic elders.

RESEARCH IMPLICATIONS

The existing data on suicide reveals wide diversity in the rates of completed suicide by each group of ethnic elders. What are the research implications?

African Americans, American Indian, and Mexican American women all have low rates of completed suicide. Clarifying the specific factors that protect these ethnic elder women from suicide would enable investigators to establish whether these factors could be applied to ethnic elder men. Further, it would be possible to see whether these factors could be identified in other groups (e.g., white elders) and whether they were protective in nonethnic elder groups.

The highest rates of completed suicide among ethnic elders were observed in older Chinese and Japanese both resulting from the Asian Exclusion Acts. If the absence of the traditional family roles was a significant factor contributing to suicide by these elders, would a special program such as "Adopt a Grandparent" in which these elders would be linked with a young Asian American family with children prove a helpful alternative resource? Studying alternative models of reengaging this cohort of Asian elders is another important research area.

The diversity of completed suicide among Hispanic American men provides a unique opportunity to study the issue of acculturation. Puerto Rican men and Mexican American men have higher rates of completed suicide than Cuban American men. Both Puerto Rican and Mexican American elders can return to their home country with relative ease, an option not readily available to Cuban elders. A fertile area for research would be to investigate the extent to which these elders have adjusted to or not adjusted to a bicultural environment and the identification of associated levels of resulting stress related to suicidal ideation, suicide attempts, and completed suicide. As discussed, Puerto Rican suicide may relate to a failure to adapt to U.S. urban versus Puerto Rican rural culture; whereas Mexican American men who have a higher level of acculturation were found to have higher rates of phobias, anxiety disorders, and alcoholism. Studying the level of acculturation across three-generational families and the presence of completed suicide, suicide attempts, and psychopathology would be a difficult, but important, study design. With the increase in African Caribbean elders in the African-origin U.S. population and the potential increase in ethnic European immigrants because of the political changes in Eastern Europe and Russia, the effect of level of acculturation and its meaning for various groups of ethnic elders is a crucial area of research.

The virtual absence of data on American Indian suicide, especially intertribal differences, should encourage epidemiologists, psychiatrists, and social scientists to identify the specific factors in given tribal groups that are protective against or at risk for completed suicide. How these factors relate to those found in other groups of ethnic elders as well as to older white men at higher risk to complete suicide would be another important research question.

The role of socioeconomic class may confound the issue of level of acculturation. Cuban American elders, the current cohort, include a significant number of professionals who immigrated with the Castro Revolution. How do those Cuban elders who complete suicide differ from those who do not? Is the level of acculturation to American society the same or different? What factors are identified as protective and which factors are identified as increasing the risk to complete a suicide in these middle-class ethnic elders?

Other study questions concern future cohorts of ethnic elders. Will the rates of completed suicide for the ethnic elder of 2050 resemble or differ from the rates of white elders? As these ethnic elders will have been born in the 1960s, their cohort experience will have been significantly different than the current cohort of ethnic elders. Will the rates of completed suicide change for ethnic elder women who begin childbearing in their teenage years and may have remained a single parent with the attendant psychosocial stressors? What will be the effect of the polysubstance abuse pattern now endemic in the U.S. population on ethnic elders of 2050 in contrast to white elders of 2050? Will suicide rates become similar or remain varied depending on the specific group of ethnic elders? To what extent, if any, will the level of acculturation influence third-, fourth-, and fifth-generation ethnic elders?

These are a few of the emerging research questions regarding ethnic elder suicide as well as research questions contrasting ethnic elder suicide and suicides by older whites. To date, few investigators have pursued these studies. It is hoped that this clarification of specific research opportunities will change that status.

REFERENCES

American Psychiatric Association. (1987). *Diagnostic and statistical manual of mental disorders* (3rd ed., rev.). Washington, DC: Author.

Baker, F. M. (1982). The black elderly: Biopsychosocial perspective within an age cohort and an adult development context. *Journal of Geriatric Psychiatry, 15,* 225–237.

Baker, F. M. (1987). The Afro-American life cycle: Success, failure, and mental health. *Journal of the National Medical Association, 79,* 626–633.

Baker, F. M. (1988). Afro-Americans. In L. Comas-Diaz and E. E. H. Griffith (Eds.), *Clinical guidelines in cross-cultural mental health* (pp. 151–181). New York: Wiley.

Baker, F. M. (1989). Black youth suicide: Literature review with a focus on prevention. In M. R. Reinleib (Ed.), *Report of the secretary's task force on youth suicide: Volume III. Prevention and interventions in youth suicide* (pp. 3-177–3-195). Washington, DC: U.S. Government Printing Office.

Baker, F. M. (1990). Ethnic minority elders: Differential diagnosis, medication, treatment, and outcomes. In M. S. Harper (Ed.), *Minority aging: Essential curricula content for selected health and allied health professionals* (pp. 549–577). Washington, DC: U.S. Government Printing Office.

Baker, F. M. (1991). Dementing illness in African American populations: Evaluation and management for the primary physician. *Journal of Geriatric Psychiatry, 24,* 73–91.

Baker, F. M., Lavizzo-Mourey, R., & Jones, B. E. (in press). Acute care of the African American elder. *Journal of Geriatric Psychiatry and Neurology.*

Baker, F. M., & Lightfoot, O. D. (1995). Geriatric psychiatry: The evaluation and treatment of psychiatric disorders in ethnic elders. In A. C. Gaw (Ed.), *Culture, ethnicity, and mental illness* (pp. 55–80). Washington, DC: American Psychiatric Press.

Block, M. R. (1979). Exiled Americans: The plight of Indian aged in the United States. In D. E. Gelfand & A. J. Kutzik (Eds.), *Ethnicity and aging: Theory, research, and policy* (pp. 184–192). New York: Springer.

Brown, D. (1971). *Bury my heart at Wounded Knee—An Indian history of the American West.* New York: Holt, Rinehart and Winston.

Burnam, M. A., Hough, R. I., Karno, M. (1987). Acculturation and lifetime prevalence of psychiatric disorders among Mexican Americans in Los Angeles. *Journal of Health and Social Behavior, 28,* 80–102.

Bush, J. S. (1976). Suicide and blacks: A conceptual framework. *Suicide and Life-Threatening Behavior, 6,* 216–311.

Carter, J. H. (1988). Health attitudes/promotions/preventions: The black elderly. In J. S. Jackson (Ed.), *The black American elderly. Research on physical and psychosocial health* (pp. 292–302). New York: Springer.

Clevenger, J. (1982). Native Americans. In A. Gaw (Ed.), *Cross-cultural psychiatry* (pp. 149–158). Boston: John Wright.

Comer, J. P. (1973). Black suicide: A hidden crisis. *Urban Health, 2,* 41–44.

Cuellar, J. (1990a). *Aging and health: American Indian/Alaskan Native* (SGEC Working Paper Series, Number 6, Ethnogeriatric Reviews). Stanford, CA: Stanford Geriatric Education Center.

Cuellar, J. (1990b). *Aging and health: Hispanic American elder* (SGEC Working Paper Series, Number 5, Ethnogeriatric Reviews). Stanford, CA: Stanford Geriatric Education Center.

Cuellar, J. B., Stanford, E. P., & Miller-Soule, D. J. (1982). *Understanding minority aging: Perspectives and sources.* San Diego: San Diego State University, University Center on Aging.

Davis, R. (1980). Suicide among young blacks: Trends and perspectives. *Phylon, 41,* 223–229.

Dressler, W. W., & Bernal, H. (1982). Acculturation and stress in a low income Puerto Rican community. *Journal of Human Stress, 8,* 32–38.

Durkheim, E. (1951). *Suicide: A study in sociology.* New York: Free Press.

Escobar, J. L., Burnam, A., Karno, M. (1986). Use of the Mini-Mental State Examination (MMSE) in a community population of mixed ethnicity: Cultural and linguistic artifacts. *Journal of Nervous and Mental Disease, 174,* 607–614.

Fellin, P. A., & Powell, T. J. (1988). Mental health services and older adult minorities: An assessment. *Gerontologist, 28,* 442–447.

Griffith, E. E. H., & Bell, C. C. (1989). Recent trends in suicide and homicide among blacks. *Journal of the American Medical Association, 262,* 2265–2269.

Griffith, E. E. H., & Delgado, A. K., Foulks, E., Ruiz, P., Spiegel, J., Wintrob, R., & Yamamoto, J. (1989a). *Group for the Advancement of Psychiatry: Report No. 128. Suicide and ethnicity in the United States.* New York: Brunner/Mazel.

Griffith, E. E. H., & Delgado, A. K., Foulks, E., Ruiz, P., Spiegel, J., Wintrob, R., & Yamamoto, J. (1989b). Suicide among blacks in the United States. In E. E. H. Griffith, A. K. Delgado, & E. Foulks, et al., *Group for the Advancement of Psychiatry: Report No. 128. Suicide and ethnicity in the United States* (pp. 11–29). New York: Brunner/Mazel.

Griffith, E. E. H., & Delgado, A. K., Foulks, E., Ruiz, P., Spiegel, J., Wintrob, R., & Yamamoto, J. (1989c). Suicide among American Indians and Alaskan Natives. In E. E. H. Griffith, A. K. Delgado, & E. Foulks, et al., *Group for the Advancement of Psychiatry: Report No. 128. Suicide and ethnicity in the United States* (pp. 30–57). New York: Brunner/Mazel.

Griffith, E. E. H., & Delgado, A. K., Foulks, E., Ruiz, P., Spiegel, J., Wintrob, R., & Yamamoto, J. (1989d). Suicide among the Chinese and Japanese. In E. E. H. Griffith, A. K. Delgado, & E. Foulks, et al., *Group for the Advancement of Psychiatry: Report No. 128. Suicide and ethnicity in the United States* (pp. 58–71). New York: Brunner/Mazel.

Griffith, E. E. H., & Delgado, A. K., Foulks, E., Ruiz, P., Spiegel, J., Wintrob, R., & Yamamoto, J. (1989e). Suicide among Hispanic Americans. In E. E. H. Griffith, A. K. Delgado, & E. Foulks, et al., *Group for the*

Advancement of Psychiatry: Report No. 128. Suicide and ethnicity in the United States (pp. 72–94). New York: Brunner/Mazel.

Griffith, E. E. H., & Delgado, A. K., Foulks, E., Ruiz, P., Spiegel, J., Wintrob, R., & Yamamoto, J. (1989f). Summary and discussion. In E. E. H. Griffith, A. K. Delgado, & E. Foulks, et al., *Group for the Advancement of Psychiatry: Report No. 128. Suicide and ethnicity in the United States* (pp. 95–113). New York: Brunner/Mazel.

Harper, M. S. (Ed.). (1990). *Minority aging: Essential curricula content for selected health and allied health professions* (DHHS Publication No. HRS P-DV-90-4). Washington, DC: U.S. Government Printing Office.

Hendin, H. (1969). Black suicide. *Archives of General Psychiatry, 21,* 401–422.

Henry, A. F., & Short, J. F. (1954). *Suicide and homicide.* New York: Free Press.

Hoppe, S. K., & Martin, H. W. (1986). Patterns of suicide among Mexican Americans and Anglos, 1960–1980. *Social Psychiatry, 21,* 83–88.

John, R. (1991, April). *Setting a research agenda on American Indian aging.* Special paper prepared for the Gerontological Society of America, Task Force on Minority Issues in gerontology. Warrenton, VA: Arlie House.

Kemp, B. J., Staples, F., & Lopez-Aqueres, W. (1987). Epidemiology of depression and dysphoria in an elderly Hispanic population: Prevalence and correlates. *Journal of the American Geriatrics Society, 35,* 920–926.

King, L. M. (1982). Suicide from a "black reality" perspective. In B. A. Bass, G. E. Wyatt, & G. J. Powell (Eds.), *The Afro-American family: Assessment, treatment, and research issues* (pp. 221–236). New York: Grune & Stratton.

Lacuyo, C. G. (1980). Hispanics. In E. B. Palmore (Ed.), *Handbook of the aged in the United States* (pp. 253–267). Westport, CT: Greenwood Press.

Liu, W., & Yu, E. (1985). Ethnicity, mental health, and the urban delivery system. In J. Maldorodo & J. Moore (Eds.), *Urban ethnicity in the United States* (pp. 211–247). Beverly Hills: Sage.

Longino, C. F., & Smith, K. J. (1991). Black retirement migration in the United States. *Journal of Gerontology, 46,* S125–S132.

Manson, S. M., & Callaway, D. (1988). Health and aging among American Indians: Issues and challenges for the biobehavioral sciences. In S. M. Manson & N. Dinges (Eds.), *Health and behavior: A research agenda for American Indians* (pp. 160–210). Denver: University of Colorado Health Sciences Center.

Manson, S. M., Shore, J. H., & Bloom, J. D. (1985). The depressive experience in American Indian communities: A challenge for psychiatric theory and diagnosis. In A. Kleinman & B. Good (Eds.), *Culture and depression* (pp. 331–368). Berkeley: University of California Press.

Manson, S. M., Walker, R. D., & Kivlahan, D. R. (1987). Psychiatric assessment and treatment of American Indians and Alaskan Natives. *Hospital and Community Psychiatry, 38,* 165–173.

Maris, R. W. (1969). *Social forces in urban suicide.* Homewood, IL: Dorsey Press.

Markides, K. S. (1986). Minority status, aging, and mental health. *International Journal of Aging and Human Development, 23,* 285–300.

Markides, K. S., & Mindel, C. H. (1987). *Aging and ethnicity.* Beverly Hills: Sage.

Martinez, C. (1988). Mexican Americans. In *Clinical guidelines in cross-cultural mental health* (pp. 182–203). New York: Wiley.

Matsugi, N. (1980). *Tokyo shimbun.* Phoenix: Asian Foundation.

McIntosh, J. L., & Santos, J. F. (1985–1986). Methods of suicide by age: Sex and race differences among the young and old. *International Journal of Aging and Human Development, 22,* 123–139.

Mercer, S. O. (1989). *Elder suicide: A national survey of prevention and intervention programs.* Washington, DC: American Association of Retired Persons.

Miller, M. (1971). Suicides on a southwestern American Indian reservation. *White Cloud Journal, 1,* 14–18.

Monk, M., & Warshauer, M. E. (1974). Completed and attempted suicide in three ethnic groups. *American Journal of Epidemiology, 100,* 333–345.

Morioka-Douglas, N., & Yeo, G. (1990). *Aging and health: Asian/Pacific Island American Elders* (SGEC Working Paper Series, No. 3, Ethnogeriatric Reviews). Stanford, CA: Stanford Geriatric Education Center.

National Center for Health Statistics. (1991). *Health. United States, 1990.* Hyattsville, MD: U.S. Public Health Service.

Pine, C. (1981). Suicide: American Indian and Alaskan Native tradition. *White Cloud Journal, 2,* 3–8.

Prudhomme, G., & Musto, D. F. (1973). Historical perspective on mental health and racism in the United States. In C. V. Willie, B. M. Kramer, & K. B. S. Brown (Eds.), *Racism and mental health* (pp. 25–57). Pittsburgh: University of Pittsburgh Press.

Richardson, J. (1990). *Aging and health: Black American Elders* (SGEC Working Paper Series, No. 4, Ethnogeriatric Reviews). Stanford, CA: Stanford Geriatric Education Center.

Rosenthal, M. P., Goldfarb, N. J., Carlson, B. L., Sagi, P. C. & Balaban, D. J. (1987). Assessment of depression in a family practice center. *Journal of Family Practice, 25,* 143–149.

Sakauye, K. M., Baker, F. M., Chacko, R. C., Jimenez, R. G., Nickeus, H. W., Thompson, J. W., de Figueiredo, J. M., Liu, W., & Manson, S. (1995). *Report of the Task Force on Ethnic Minority Elderly.* Washington, DC: American Psychiatric Association.

Salcido, R. M., Nakano, C., & Jue, S. (1980). The use of formal and informal health and welfare services of the Asian-American elderly. *California Sociologist, 3,* 213–229.

Seiden, R. H. (1981). Mellowing with age. Factors influencing the nonwhite suicide rate. *Journal of Aging and Human Development, 13,* 265–284.

Smith, J. C., Mercy, J. A., & Warren, C. W. (1985). Hispanic suicide: Report for five southwestern states for the years 1976–1980. *Suicide and Life-Threatening Behavior, 1,* 14–26.

U.S. Bureau of the Census. (1988). Population Data. Washington, DC: U.S. Government Printing Office.

Van Winkle, N., & May, P. (1986). Native American suicide in New Mexico, 1957–1979: A comparative study. *Human Organization, 45,* 296–309.

Warshauer, M. E., & Monk, M. (1978). Problems in suicide statistics for whites and blacks. *American Journal of Public Health, 68,* 383–388.

Westermeyer, J. (1979). Disorganization: Its role in Indian suicide rates. *American Journal of Psychiatry, 128,* 123–129.

Worobey, J. L., & Hogan, D. P. (1991, April). *The demography of minority aging populations.* Special paper prepared for the Gerontological Society of America, Task Force on Minority Issues in Gerontology. Warrenton, VA: Arlie House.

Wykle, M., & Kaskel, B. (1991, April). Research agenda for increasing the longevity of minority older adults through improved health status. Special paper prepared for the Gerontological Society of America, Task Force on Minority Issues in Gerontology. Warrenton, VA: Arlie House.

Wylie, F. M. (1971). Attitudes toward aging and the aged among black Americans: Some historical perspectives. *Aging and Human Development, 2,* 66–70.

Yamamoto, J. (1976). Japanese American suicide in Los Angeles. In J. Westermeyer (Ed.), *Anthropology and mental health* (pp. 29–36). Chicago: Moutan.

PART II
Therapeutic Approaches

5

Clinical Measurement of Suicidality and Coping in Late Life
A Theory of Countervailing Forces

ROBERT PLUTCHIK,
ALEXANDER J. BOTSIS,
MARCELLA BAKUR WEINER, AND
GARY J. KENNEDY

In this chapter, we examine problems of using standard scales for measuring depression or suicidality. Because we believe that suicidality is the result of an interaction between life stressors and individual coping styles, we will also consider the nature of coping. We present a theory of coping, a measure of coping styles, and some insights obtained through its use. Finally, a number of comments are made on the issue of treatment of suicidality in the elderly.

RISK FACTORS FOR SUICIDE IN THE ELDERLY

Suicidal behavior is difficult to predict. Even in high-risk groups, it is infrequent, and the base rate of suicide in the general population is low.

Therefore, even "good" predictor variables will identify many false positives. Another reason for the difficulty in prediction is that many different variables contribute in some degree to the probability of suicidal behavior. Each variable makes only a small contribution to the likelihood of action, and thus each affects the threshold for overt behavior in unpredictable ways (Plutchik, van Praag, & Conte, 1989a).

However, studies of attempted and completed suicides among the elderly suggest that a number of factors aid the clinician in determining suicide risk. Darbonne (1969) analyzing 259 suicide notes cited illness, pain, physical disability, loneliness, and isolation as reasons for suicide among the elderly. Based on his studies of completed suicides of elderly males, Miller (1976) concluded that late-life suicide may be classified into one of the following eight patterns:

1. Reaction to physical illness.
2. Reaction to mental illness.
3. Reaction to retirement.
4. Reaction to death of a spouse.
5. Reaction to threat of dependency or institutionalization.
6. Pathological personal relationships.
7. Alcoholism and drug abuse.
8. Some combination of these factors.

The following subsections briefly review physical health problems, depression, alcoholism, dementia and other risk factors for suicide. We conclude with a description of a countervailing forces theory of suicide to define the interrelationships of the many variables that either increase or decrease the risk of suicide.

Physical Health Problems

According to Barraclough (1971), the onset of significant illness strongly increases the risk of suicide. Sainsbury (1962) has reported that physical illness preceded 35% of suicides of older persons. Miller (1976) reported that 62% of the suicides of elderly white males he studied were the result of physical illness. Dorpat, Anderson, and Ripley (1968) found that, of the 60 completed suicides they studied, 70% of the subjects suffered from some illness.

The aged suffer from chronic, debilitating diseases, such as cancer, Parkinson's disease, arthritis, heart disease, and stroke. Among the many consequences of such diseases are pain and suffering, disfigurement, anxiety, worry, depression, loss of self-confidence, interruption of significant life activities and altered interpersonal relationships. Illness results in physical stress on the aged body, which due to physiological changes accompanying the aging process, is less able to endure such stress. Based on their reviews of several studies, Cohen and Lazarus (1979) suggest that illness poses threats to life, threats to bodily comfort and integrity, threats to one's emotional equilibrium, threats to self-concept and future plans, and threats to the fulfillment of customary social roles and activities in work, the family, and the community.

Depression

Psychiatric disorders represent an important risk factor for suicide among the elderly. Depression is one of the two most common psychiatric disorders of old age, yet its prevalence, incidence, and nature remain controversial (Blazer, 1980). Although depression has been clearly established as a risk factor for suicide in younger adults, there is relatively little information on this issue in the elderly (Guze & Robins, 1970; Plutchik, van Praag, & Conte, 1989a; Pokorny, 1983).

On the other hand, according to Batchelor (1957), at least 80% of suicidal elderly suffer from depression. Capstick (1960) found the prevalence of depression in cases of late-life suicide to be approximately 48%, whereas O'Neal, Robins, and Shmidt (1956) cited a higher rate (70%) of depressive symptoms among those elderly who attempt or commit suicide.

In addition, Guze and Robins (1970) estimated that the lifetime risk of suicide was approximately 15% for persons with primary affective disorders; and Jamison (1979) reported that among patients with unipolar or bipolar affective disorders the suicide risk is higher for those whose clinical picture is accompanied by agitation than those who have a clinical picture of retarded depression. Moreover, Payne (1975) reported that depressed older adults are more likely to attempt suicide and that their affective disorders are often not appropriately diagnosed and treated. Nevertheless, even though depression is usually misdiagnosed and missed for several reasons among this age group, this psychopathological dimension continues to be the most common factor precipitating both attempted and completed suicides (Blazer, Bacher, & Mantom, 1986).

Alcoholism

Increased rates of suicide are associated with problem drinking among the elderly, especially in those with primary and affective disorders (Schuckit & Miller, 1976). Gardner, Bahn, and Mack (1964) reported that 17% of older persons with known psychiatric contact who committed suicide had a history of alcoholism. Schuckit and Pastor (1978, 1979) noted that late-onset alcoholism is more strongly associated with suicide. However, elderly alcoholics both early and late onset have a higher suicide rate than nonalcoholics. Alcoholism may interact with other risk factors as well.

Although the evidence on the issue is controversial, in terms of prevalence alcoholism is, next to cognitive impairment, probably the most common diagnosable mental disorder of later life (Osgood & Thielman, 1990). It has long been noted that alcoholism and depression are seen in the same individuals (Amark, 1951). Rates of depression among alcoholics have been reported to vary between 3% and 98% (Keeler, Taylor, & Miller, 1979), with the results of the majority of studies ranging between 30% and 60% (Bowen et al., 1984).

Cook, Winokur, Garvey, and Beach (1991) suggested that depressed male elderly patients with a past history of alcoholism differ from depressives without such a history. According to Cook et al., such subjects appear to present more frequently with a chronic reactive-type of depression. Features of "neurotic-reactive" depression as outlined by Winokur (1985) appear to persist in this group of elderly depressives with a history of alcoholism. Such features include frequent readmission to hospital, more chronic continuation of antidepressant medications, more suicidal ideation, and less frequent remission of depressive symptoms.

Dementia

Dementia occurs in up to 20% of people over 65 (Gruenberg, 1978) and is the leading cause of admission into nursing facilities. The most common cause of dementia is Alzheimer's disease, which accounts for about 60% of all cases of dementia (Terry & Katzman, 1983). Although cognitive impairment is characteristic of the dementias, it is not diagnostic of them, since it appears in many psychiatric disorders including depression (pseudodementia).

Other Factors

Social isolation has repeatedly been associated with suicide in old age. Barraclough (1971) found that isolation had the highest correlation with suicide compared with any other social variable. Bereavement has also been associated with suicide among the elderly (MacMahon & Pugh, 1965). The relatively high rate of suicide among widows, particularly in the first year of widowhood, suggests that what is most important is the immediate loss of a spouse rather than the isolated state itself. Paykel, Prusoff, and Myers (1975) found that 21% of the elderly who committed suicide had reported bereavement within 6 months prior to the suicide, compared with 4% of a group of matched controls. Finally, the risk for future suicidal behavior is increased if an individual has a history of previous gestures or suicide attempts (Plutchik & van Praag, 1990).

A Theory of Countervailing Forces in Suicide

Do we need a theory of suicide for the elderly that is different from that used to describe other age groups? There are some average differences between the elderly and younger adults, but that does not mean we need two different theories. In the same sense, although men have different suicide rates from women and blacks have different rates from whites, we do not require separate theories of suicide for women and for African Americans.

In an effort to develop a general model to help understand the nature of suicide in all groups, Plutchik et al. (1989a) have developed a two-stage model of countervailing forces. The two-stage model of countervailing forces (Plutchik et al., 1989a; Plutchik & van Praag, 1990) assumes that any behavior is a vectorial resultant of the interaction of opposing forces. According to this model, a relatively small number of triggers generate aggressive impulses. The major triggers are threats, challenges, insults, loss of control, and decreases in one's perceived hierarchical position (Blanchard & Blanchard, 1984). The aggressive impulse generated by these triggers may then be amplified or attenuated, depending on the presence or absence of other factors. Variables that act as amplifiers include physical symptoms, mental illness, loss of significant others, severe illness, poor coping styles, and access to weapons. Variables that may serve as attenuators include having a family network, certain coping styles, and certain personality traits (e.g., timidity) (Pfeffer, Plutchik, & Misruchi, 1983; Plutchik, Climent, & Ervin, 1976). Because both amplifying and attenuating factors coexist at any one time, the strength of the aggressive impulse will be a vectorial resultant of the presence of these opposing or countervailing forces. This balancing process, which is called the Stage I vectorial summation, determines the level of the aggressive impulse that is acted on as suicidal behavior.

Action, however, requires an object toward which it is directed. Depression, a large number of life problems (including work, medical, and family problems), feelings of hopelessness, and recent psychiatric symptoms are among the factors that predispose an individual to direct the aggressive impulse toward the self, resulting in a risk of suicide. In contrast, the trait of impulsivity, problems with the civil or criminal justice system, and recent life stresses all dispose the individual to direct the aggressive impulse toward others, resulting in a risk of violence. These two sets of variables that determine the goal of the aggressive impulse are referred to as Stage II of the model of countervailing forces. Figure 5–1 describes a schematic representation of the model.

The specific variables that act as either amplifiers or attenuators must be determined by clinical research and by clinical experience. It is quite possible that the relative importance of certain variables will be greater or less in an elderly population. It is also conceivable that a few variables may operate primarily in the elderly just as a few other variables may operate primarily in adolescents.

At present, the data are scanty but we can propose hypotheses based on clinical experience about salient amplifiers and attenuators of suicide risk in the elderly. Some possible amplifiers are:

- Severe physical illness.
- Marked change of body image.
- Loss of significant emotional ties.
- Decrease in level of socialization.
- Lack of a religious faith.
- Physical disability.
- Cognitive deficiencies.
- Changing of loss of familiar surroundings.
- Isolation.
- Loss of functional capacities.
- Chronic pain.
- Reduction of responsibilities.

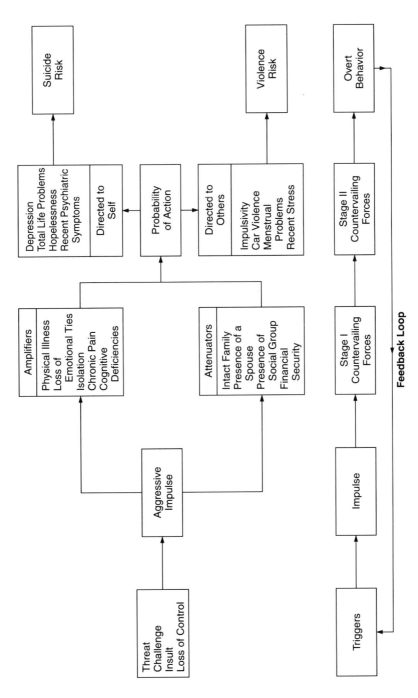

Figure 5-1. Two-stage model of suicide and violence.

89

- Reduction in sense of value or usefulness within society and within family.

Some possible attenuators are:

- Intact and close-knit family.
- Adequate medical care.
- Sense of financial security.
- Presence of a spouse.
- Presence of a social group.
- Continuing opportunity for useful work.
- Continuing sexual life.

We want to emphasize that these lists represent hypotheses that may be used to guide future research. It should be possible to empirically determine whether each of these variables do in fact operate as amplifiers or attenuators and also to determine the relative influence on the risk of suicide. It is our belief that well-established variables such as depression, hopelessness, marital conflict, psychiatric illness and so on, operate within the elderly just as they do in younger people. If these hypotheses turn out to be correct they can be used in connection with the psychotherapy of distressed elderly people. This point will be elaborated in a later section.

ASSESSING SUICIDALITY IN THE ELDERLY

Psychological factors play a crucial part in late life suicide. The elderly suffer many losses, including loss of health; impaired vision and hearing; loss of mobility; financial loss; loss of home and possessions; loss of independence; cognitive slowing and impairment; and loss of social roles in work, family, and the community. These losses result in stress at a time in life when the individual is least able to cope with stress. And the stress suffered as a consequence often results in feelings of loneliness, hopelessness, helplessness, and depression. Many older individuals experience a deep sense of emptiness and meaninglessness and lose all motivation for working, playing, and even living. Despite this grim picture, it should be emphasized that a number of positive elements are associated with the aging process. These may include a decrease in responsibilities, an increase in knowledge, an increase in self-acceptance, and an increase in wisdom.

Measuring Depression

Depression is a well-established correlate of suicide attempts and completions. However, the true incidence of depression among the elderly is controversial. Data vary from study to study and seem to depend on where an investigation was conducted (at an inpatient or an outpatient facility or in the general population; Kennedy et al., 1989).

Psychiatric epidemiologists have approached the problem by surveying the general population for depressive symptoms. Not surprisingly, a different picture emerges from this effort. Boyd et al. (1982) have demonstrated that at any given time a majority of the U.S. population has one or two depressive symptoms. Indeed, between 9% and 20% of the population have enough symptoms to score in the "depressed range" on self-report symptom scales. In geriatric population surveys, rates of significant depressive symptoms in the elderly, estimated by using symptom checklists, range from 10% to 45%. However, studies using clinical psychiatric evaluations have indicated that the prevalence of major depression or dysthymia in the older population is only between 2% and 5% (Blazer, 1982). These studies would seem to indicate that, although the prevalence of diagnosable depression is not much greater in the elderly than in the general population, the group of elderly people who suffer significant depressive symptoms may indeed be larger.

Furthermore, if we consider that the elderly do not frequently complain of depression or sadness but rather focus on physical complaints, worries, or family and financial problems and also present with cognitive dysfunction that is too quickly ascribed to a dementia, our ability to assess depression will be more difficult. Approximately 12% of the elderly diagnosed as suffering from a dementia are thought to actually have a pseudodementia resulting from undiagnosed and untreated depression (Addonizio & Shamoian, 1986).

To complicate the matter further, the validity of existing self-report measures of depression with elderly subjects has recently been questioned. Several studies indicate that the pattern of response to such measures by elderly subjects is distorted by the overlap between typical depressive symptomatology and changes associated with the aging process itself. They also suggest that age produces a differential pattern of response to such questionnaires, with the somatic symptoms being preferentially responded to, whereas emotional-psychological symptoms are underreported (Oltman, Michals, & Steer, 1980).

Because of these problems, evaluation of any older person frequently requires an interview with the individual's family and/or supporting figures as well as the testing and evaluation of the patient. Unfortunately, there are as yet no unequivocal tests to differentiate pseudodementia from dementia. The diagnosis of pseudodementia is currently based on the patient's history, the physician's clinical observation, and the patient's therapeutic response to antidepressant treatment. Useful clinical criteria for the diagnosis of pseudodementia have been reported by Wells (1979).

Measuring Suicidality

Any attempt to measure suicide risk in the elderly should be based on general methods for measuring suicide risk in any other population. Suicide risk scales are generally constructed by defining a number of variables that are believed on the basis of empirical research or clinical judgment to be related to suicide risk. High scores obtained on such instruments are then presumed to provide an index of suicidehrisk. This index then needs to be subjected to other criteria of validation.

Our review of the literature has not revealed this kind of suicide risk scale specifically directed for use with the elderly. However, in view of the points we have made earlier concerning the basic continuity of risk factors in all age groups, it is reasonable to assume that suicide risk scales developed in younger populations may be useful in the geriatric population.

One such measure is the Suicide Risk Scale (SRS) developed by Plutchik, van Praag, and Conte (1989b). It consists of 15 items that have been cross-validated with several psychiatric populations as a discriminator of patients with and without a history of suicide attempts. Sensitivity and specifically are reasonably high, and we believe it may serve as a useful research tool in studies of the elderly. Table 5–1 displays the items of the scale.

ISSUES OF COPING

All people face the challenges of physical decline, illness, loss of friends, decreased sexual interest and capacity as they get older. To age successfully, people have to use coping styles that were effective in the past, or learn to develop new mechanisms for adapting to these stressful situations.

TABLE 5–1
Suicide Risk Scale

Name_____ Date_____ Age_____
Sex_____ Clinical Service_____

Instructions

The following questions are about things that you have felt or done. Please answer each question with a simple Yes or No.

	Yes	No
1. Do you take drugs such as aspirin or sleeping pills regularly?	___	___
2. Do you have trouble falling asleep?	___	___
3. Do you sometimes feel that you will lose control of yourself?	___	___
4. Do you have little interest in being with people?	___	___
5. Do you feel that your future will be more unpleasant than pleasant?	___	___
6. Do you ever feel you are worthless?	___	___
7. Do you feel hopeless about your future?	___	___
8. Do you often feel so frustrated, that you just want to lie down and quit struggling altogether?	___	___
9. Do you feel depressed now?	___	___
10. Are you separated, divorced or widowed?	___	___
11. Has anyone in your family ever tried to commit suicide?	___	___
12. Have you ever been so angry that you felt you might kill someone?	___	___
13. Have you ever thought about committing suicide?	___	___
14. Have you ever told anyone you would commit suicide?	___	___
15. Have you ever tried to kill yourself?	___	___

Several studies addressing the question of age-related differences in coping styles found decreases in the use of what might be considered "adaptive" coping mechanisms. Quayhagen and Quayhagen (1982), for example, found age differences in responses on three factors of their Coping Strategies Inventory: affectivity, problem solving, and help-seeking. Their oldest group (mean age 66.6) scored higher on affectivity (use of emotional expression) and lower on problem-solving. There was a linear decrease in help-seeking across all age groups. Cicirelli (1989) also reported a decrease in help-seeking strategies for his elderly sample. Cohen

(1980) interviewed older people just before their surgery and categorized coping styles as avoidant and vigilant. He reported a positive correlation between age and frequency of using avoidant coping strategies. Sadly, suicide may be the ultimate in avoidant coping.

The literature reveals decreases in the number of coping mechanisms older people use. However, some studies suggest an age-related decrease in adaptive coping styles, whereas others suggest an age-related decrease in maladaptive coping styles (Meeks, Carstensen, Tamsky, Wright, & Pellegrini, 1989). Thus, age-related differences in coping emerge with reasonable consistency: There are quantifiable changes in coping activity with age. The exact nature and significance of these differences, however, remain unclear.

The literature on coping in the elderly is to some degree confusing because of different conceptual frameworks, a lack of explicit definitions, and the use of different methods of measurement. For these reasons, we propose a conceptualization of coping that has been found to be useful and may serve to guide research in this area of suicidology (Conte, Plutchik, Picard, Galanter, & Jacoby, 1991; Plutchik, 1989; Plutchik & Conte, 1989).

During the past several decades, the senior author of this chapter has been developing a general psychoevolutionary theory of emotions (Plutchik, 1970, 1980a, 1980b, 1990). This theory has many interrelated concepts. It assumes that emotions are more than feelings states, facial expressions, or physiological changes. Emotions are complex chains of events triggered by certain stimuli. They involve cognitive interpretations, feelings states, physiological changes, impulses to action, display behavior, and overt action designed to modify the initial triggering stimuli. The psychoevolutionary theory of emotion is based on a number of explicit postulates (Plutchik, 1980a). The postulate most relevant to the concept of coping styles is that emotions are related to a number of derivative conceptual domains. This assumes that one may use different "languages" to describe aspects of emotion, and that these languages are related to one another in systematic ways.

According to the psychoevolutionary theory, coping styles are the conscious derivatives of the unconscious ego defenses. For example, the unconscious defense of denial corresponds to the conscious coping style of "minimization." The ego defense of displacement corresponds to the coping style of "substitution," and the defense of intellectualization corresponds to the coping style of "mapping." It is possible to define a small number (eight) of basic coping styles that are related to the basic emotions (eight) and that have applicability to life problems including the threat of suicide. The eight coping styles will be briefly described both as risk-increasing and risk-decreasing language.

Mapping

One way that individuals deal with problems is by using their innate curiosity and intelligence to get more information about the problem. If a person went to a physician and described headaches, a rash, and a slight fever, the physician would probably ask for more information about feelings, and symptoms, and do blood tests, X rays, and other evaluations. In a sense, doctors expand their understanding of an illness by making a map of the territory, by getting to know as much as possible about the situation. Only then can physicians make an educated judgment designed to diagnose the problem and suggest the best solution.

In the same sense, a person needs as much information as possible about a problem before taking actions to deal with it. If a woman were to discover in her elderly mother's room some expensive items of jewelry, mapping would imply that she find out (a) if these are in fact newly purchased, (b) if she is handling them for someone else, (c) if these were borrowed from someone else, or (d) if they were stolen. Only after obtaining such information would she be in a position to act appropriately. Mapping means trying to cope with a problem by getting more information about it. However mapping out the means of suicide is clear preparation for self-destruction, and, as we will demonstrate, an awareness of the purpose to which a given coping style is put is an essential step on assessing suicide risk.

Avoidance

Another way to deal with a problem is by avoiding the situation that gives rise to the problem. If there is someone who is difficult to get along with, it may be possible to avoid any contact with that person. Many older people who cannot tolerate cold weather relocate to warmer climates. Older people also tend to be more selective of their friends and avoid people who are critical or difficult to be with.

Help-Seeking

Another way to solve problems is to ask for help. Sometimes help-seeking is carried out on a very informal basis. For example, older people may call on friends, neighbors, and relatives when they are ill. Sometimes difficult life problems may require help-seeking from an expert. For example, elderly people may see doctors frequently or join a support group.

Minimizing

Many situations are ambiguous in their implications—any individual and different people can interpret the same situation in different or even opposite ways (the glass-half-full optimist or half-empty pessimist). The objective facts are the same, but the emotion felt depends on how the person interprets the facts. Minimization refers to the idea that individuals can minimize the importance or seriousness of events in their life and then can choose this method of coping as a conscious strategy.

In studies of middle managers in a large national corporation, it was found that those managers who tended to minimize problems experienced less stress on the job and were still rated as good managers (Bunker, 1982). Many older people tend to minimize the severity of their illnesses or dysfunctions to bolster their sense of cohesiveness and confidence. Thus, older patients may be allowed to minimize the danger of suicidal thought, but their family and care providers should not.

Reversal

This idea refer to the coping style that leads individuals to do the opposite of what they feel. Such behavior is not a sign of hypocrisy but is frequently a socially effective way of handling certain problems.

In many ways, acceptable social behavior depends on people acting in ways opposite to their feelings. The ideas of politeness, tact, graciousness, and diplomacy all relate to people acting differently than they feel. Many elderly people are asked by their grown children to baby-sit. Despite reluctance to do so, they seldom decline the invitation in order to maintain social and emotional family ties. In contrast, casual mention of suicidal ideas will serve to mobilize others to attempt reversal. And repeated denials of suicidal thought call for inquiry into just what is being served by the denials.

Blame

Some people cope with problems by blaming other people. This method works well under certain conditions, at least for a while. It makes the person doing the blaming feel good because he or she does not take responsibility for the problem. In modern life, we all are faced with the problem of completing forms and questionnaires. When older people find such tasks difficult to do, they may tend to blame the forms or form makers as responsible for the difficulties.

Placing blame on a person or situation helps the blamer feel a little better, but it does not solve the problem. Blaming makes the person being blamed feel bad, with the strong likelihood that the blamed person will develop resentment. Resentment, in turn, tends to lead to a desire for revenge starting the vicious cycle of blame-resentment-revenge. Therefore, although blaming others helps the person cope with a problem in the short run, the long-run consequences are undesirable. Blaming others for one's suicidal thoughts may very well precipitate an invitation for a suicidal act.

Substitution

Sometimes life creates problems for which there are no direct solutions. Substitution refers to indirect methods of coping. Older people generally have limited mobility. As a result, they cope by developing hobbies and interests that can be done at home or nearby. In one survey, older people were found to describe reading, TV viewing, and visiting neighbors as primary recreational activities (Ginsberg, 1981). Other activities included gardening, walking, or dining out. All these would be substituting pleasant, enjoyable activities for more vigorous ones that may have been performed earlier or—for those on limited incomes—that required large expenditures. An inability to find substitutions for the inevitable losses in life may leave the older adult with suicide as an option.

Improving Shortcomings

Sometimes a problem is created by the person's own weaknesses. When a problem exists, many people tend to focus on how others are handling things poorly. However, it is also possible for people to look at themselves more closely and consider their own contribution to the problem. Many older people have difficulty remembering things and cope with this problem by writing notes and reminders to themselves.

Shortcomings may sometimes be in the person's own personality or attitudes. Arguments with friends or relatives may reflect a lack of tolerance or acceptance of another person's idiosyncrasies. Learning to be more accepting may go a long way toward overcoming the friction. Similarly accepting and when possible, overcoming a shortcoming is essentially antithetical to considering suicide.

These coping styles have been used in several research studies (Plutchik, 1989; Rim, 1987, 1990) and have been structured into a self-report questionnaire that provides measures of a tendency to use each of these coping styles in one's life. A study by Weiner, Plutchik, and Rubino (1991) has demonstrated that normally functioning elderly people tend to use the same coping styles as the younger adults who have provided the norms for the AECOM Coping Styles Test. Men were generally not significantly different from women on the use of the various coping styles. However, a tendency to use blame as a coping style and help-seeking as a coping style correlated significantly with the number of life problems.

The test lends itself to further research in this important area of coping in the elderly. The characterization of these styles also lends itself to clinical application both in exploring the older person's risk as well as supporting the more protective aspects of an individual's style. Knowledge of the suicidal person's coping styles helps the clinician tip the scales toward survival.

THERAPEUTIC IMPLICATIONS

Life stress is clearly dependent on the relationship between the individual and the environment. When stress becomes overwhelming, it is because the individual appraises his or her life problems as being unmanageable or as exceeding available resources. When that happens, an individual's sense of survival is threatened. From this point of view, the treatment of depression and suicidality in the elderly takes two forms. One is concerned with an internal sense of self, and the other is concerned with the structure of the environment.

Individual treatment should focus on a number of variables such as attitudes toward responsibility for self and others, coping styles as described in the previous section, religious faith and practice, a sense of the future, attitudes of self-acceptance with regard to changes of body image, health status, and physical appearance.

With regard to therapeutic intervention related to the environment, steps should be taken to provide physical and medical resources, adequate housing, and nutrition and companionship. Family contacts should be encouraged, isolation reduced, and formalized group activities encouraged or provided. At best, our efforts are small relative to the magnitude of the problem to be solved. However, if we can reduce to some degree the amplifiers of distress and suicidality and increase their attenuators we would be contributing to the well-being of people in the sunset of their lives.

REFERENCES

Addonizio, G., & Shamoian, C. A. (1986). Depression and dementia. In D. V. Jeste (Ed.), *Neuropsychiatric Dementia* (pp. 73–109). Washington, DC: American Psychiatric Press.

Amark, C. (1951). A study in alcoholism: Clinical, social-psychiatric and genetic investigations. *Acta Psychiatrica Scandinavica, 70*(suppl.), 1–283.

Atchley, R. C. (1980). Aging and suicide: Reflections on the quality of life. In S. G. Hyanes, M. Feinlib, J. A. Ross, & L. Stallones (Eds.), *Epidemiology of aging* (NIH Publication No. 8-962, pp. 141–161). Washington, DC: U.S. Department of Health and Human Services.

Barraclough, B. (1971). Suicide in the elderly. In D. W. K. Kay & A. Walk (Eds.), *Recent development in psychogeriatrics.* London: Headly Brothers.

Batchelor, I. R. C. (1957). Suicide in old age. In E. S. Schneidman & N. L. Farberow (Eds.), *Clues to suicide* (pp. 143–151). New York: McGraw-Hill.

Blanchard, D. C., & Blanchard, R. J. (1984). Affect and aggression: An animal model applied to human behavior. In R. J. Blanchard & D. C. Blanchard (Eds.), *Advances in the Study of Aggression* (Vol. 1). New York: Academic Press.

Blazer, D. G. (1980). The diagnosis of depression in the elderly. *Journal of American Geriatric Society, 28,* 52–58.

Blazer, D. G. (1982). *Depression in late life.* St. Louis: Mosby.

Blazer, D. G., Bachar, J. R., & Mantom, K. G. (1986). Suicide in late life: Review and commentary. *Journal of American Geriatric Society, 34,* 519–525.

Bowen, R. C., Cipywnyk, D., D'Arcy, C. (1984). Types of depression in alcoholic patients. *Canadian Medical Association Journal, 130,* 869–874.

Boyd, G. H., Weissman, M. M., Thompson, & Myers, J. K. (1982). Screening for depression in a community sample. *Archives of General Psychiatry, 39,* 1195–1200.

Bunker, K. A. (1982). *Comparisons of marketing subjects high and low in psychological symptoms* (Report No. CA 2059, p. 114). New York: American Telephone and Telegraph Co., Assessment Center.

Capstick, A. (1960). Recognition of emotional disturbance and the prevention of suicide. *British Medical Journal, 1,* 1179–1182.

Cicirelli, V. (1989). Feelings of attachment to siblings and well-being in later life. *Psychology and Aging, 4*(2), 211–216.

Cohen, C. (1980). Coping with surgery: Information, psychological preparation, and recovery. In L. W. Poon (Ed.), *Aging in the 1980s: Psychological issues.* Washington, DC: American Psychological Association.

Cohen, F., & Lazarus, R. (1979). Coping with the stress of illness. In G. Stone, F. Cohen, & N. Adler (Eds.), *Health and psychology: A handbook* (pp. 217–255). San Francisco: Jossey-Bass.

Conte, H. R., Plutchik, R., Picard, S., Galanter, M., & Jacoby, J. (1991). Sex differences in personality traits and coping styles of hospitalized alcoholics. *Journal of Studies on Alcohol, 52*(1), 26–32.

Cook, B. L., Winokur, G., Garvey, M. J., & Beach, V. (1991). Depression and previous alcoholism in the elderly. *British Journal of Psychiatry, 158,* 72–75.

Darbonne, A. R. (1969). Suicide and age. *Journal of Consulting and Clinical Psychology, 33,* 46–50.

Dorpat, T. L., Anderson, W. F., & Ripley, H. S. (1968). The relationship of physical illness to suicide. In H. L. P. Resnick (Ed.), *Suicidal behaviors: Diagnosis and management* (pp. 209–219). Boston: Little, Brown.

Gardner, E. A., Bahn, A. K., & Mack, J. (1964). Suicide and psychiatric care in the aging. *Archives of General Psychiatry, 10,* 547–553.

Ginsberg, B. (1981). *Patterns of leisure satisfaction: Attitudes of a select sample of retirees.* Unpublished doctoral dissertation, Teachers College of Columbia University.

Gruenberg, D. (1978). Epidemiology of senile dementia. In R. Katzman, R. D. Terry, & K. L. Bick (Eds.), *Alzheimer's disease: Senile dementia and related disorders* (pp. 72–84). New York: Raven Press.

Guze, S. B., & Robins, E. (1970). Suicide and primary affective disorders. *British Journal of Psychiatry, 117,* 437–438.

Jamison, K. R. (1979). Manic depressive illness in the elderly. In O. Kaplan (Ed.), *Psychopathology of aging* (pp. 79–95). New York: Academic Press.

Keeler, M. H., Taylor, C. I., & Miller, W. C. (1979). Are all recently detoxified alcoholics depressed? *American Journal of Psychiatry, 136,* 586–588.

Kennedy, G. J., Kelman, H. R., Thomas, C., Wisniewsky, W., Metz, H., & Bijur, P. (1989). Hierarchy of characteristics associated with depressive symptoms in an urban elderly sample. *American Journal of Psychiatry, 146,* 220–225.

MacMahon, B., & Pugh, T. F. (1965). Suicide in the widowed. *American Journal of Epidemiology, 81,* 23–31.

Meeks, S., Carstensen, L. L., Tamsky, B. F., Wright, T. L., & Pellegrini, D. (1989). Age differences in coping: Does less mean worse? *International Journal of Aging and Human Development, 28*(2), 127–140.

Miller, M. (1976). *Suicide among older men.* Unpublished dissertation. University of Michigan.

Oltman, A. M., Michals, T. J., & Steer, R. A. (1980). Structure of depression in older men and women. *Clinical Psychology, 36,* 672–675.

O'Neal, P., Robins, E., & Shmidt, E. H. (1956). A psychiatric study of attempted suicide in persons over 60 years of age. *Archives of Neurology and Psychiatry, 75,* 275–284.

Osgood, N. J., & Thielman, S. (1990). Geriatric suicidal behavior: Assessment and treatment. In S. J. Blumenthal, & D. J. Kupfer (Eds.), *Suicide over the life cycle: Risk factors, assessment, and treatment of suicidal patients* (pp. 341–379). Washington, DC: American Psychiatric Press.

Paykel, E. S., Prusoff, B. A., & Myers, J. K. (1975). Suicide attempts and recent life events. *Archives of General Psychiatry, 32,* 327–333.

Payne, E. J. (1975). Depression and suicide. In J. G. Howells (Ed.), *Modern perspectives in the psychiatry of old age* (pp. 290–312). New York: Brunner/Mazel.

Pfeffer, C. R., Plutchik, R., & Mizruchi, M. S. (1983). Suicidal and assaultive behavior in children: Classification, measurement, and interrelations. *American Journal of Psychiatry, 140*(2), 154–157.

Plutchik, R. (1970). Emotions, evolution and adaptive processes. In M. Arnold (Ed.), *Feelings and emotions: The Loyola symposium* (pp. 3–24). New York: Academic Press.

Plutchik, R. (1980a). *Emotions: A psychoevolutionary synthesis.* New York: Harper & Row.

Plutchik, R. (1980b). A psychoevolutionary theory of emotion. In R. Plutchik & H. Kellerman (Eds.), *Theories of emotion* (Vol. 1, pp. 3–33). New York: Academic Press.

Plutchik, R. (1984). Emotions: A general psychoevolutionary theory. In K. R. Scherer & A. Ekman (Eds.), *Approaches to emotion* (pp. 197–219). Hillsdale, NJ: Erlbaum.

Plutchik, R. (1989). Measuring emotions and their derivatives. In R. Plutchik & H. Kellerman (Eds.), *The measurement of emotions: Vol. 4,* (pp. 10–15). New York: Academic Press.

Plutchik, R. (1990). Emotions and psychotherapy: A psychoevolutionary perspective. In R. Plutchik & H. Kellerman (Eds.), *Emotions, psychotherapy and psychopathology* (Vol. 5, pp. 3–41). New York: Academic Press.

Plutchik, R., Climent, C., & Ervin, F. (1976). Research strategies for the study of human violence. In W. L. Smith & A. Kling (Eds.), *Issues in brain/behavior control.* New York: Spectrum.

Plutchik, R., & Conte, H. R. (1989). Measuring emotions and their derivatives: Personality traits, ego defenses, and coping styles. In S. Wetzler & M. Katz (Eds.), *Contemporary approaches to psychological assessment.* New York: Brunner/Mazel.

Plutchik, R., & van Praag, H. M. (1990). Psychosocial correlates of suicide and violence. In H. M. van Praag, R. Plutchik, & A. Apter (Eds.), *Violence and suicidality: Perspectives in clinical and psychobiological research* (pp. 37–65). New York: Brunner/Mazel.

Plutchik, R., van Praag, H. M., & Conte, H. R. (1989a). Correlates of suicide and violence risk: III. A two-stage model of countervailing forces. *Psychiatry Research, 28,* 215–225.

Plutchik, R., van Praag, H. M., & Conte, H. R. (1989b). Correlates of suicide and violence risk: I. The suicide risk measure. *Comprehensive Psychiatry, 30,* 296–302.

Pokorny, A. D. (1983). Prediction of suicide in psychiatric patients: Report of a prospective study. *Archives of General Psychiatry, 40,* 249–257.

Quayhagen, M. P., & Quayhagen, M. (1982). Coping with conflict: Measurement of age-related patterns. *Research on Aging, 4,* 364–377.

Rim, Y. (1987). A comparative study of two taxonomies of coping styles, personality and sex. *Personality and Individual Differences, 8,* 521–526.

Rim, Y. (1990). Social class differences in coping styles. *Personality and Individual Differences, 11,* 875–876.

Sainsbury, P. (1962). Suicide in later life. *Gerontologica Clinica, 4,* 161–170.

Sainsbury, P. (1968). Suicide and depression. *British Journal of Psychiatry, 2,* 1–13.

Schuckit, M. A., & Miller, P. L. (1976). Alcoholism in elderly men: A survey of a general medical ward. *Annals of New York Academy of Science, 273,* 558–571.

Schuckit, M. A., & Pastor, P. A. (1978). The elderly as a unique population. *Alcoholism, 2,* 31–38.

Schuckit, M. A., & Pastor, P. A. (1979). Alcohol related psychopathology in the aged. In O. J. Kaplan (Ed.), *Psychopathology of aging* (pp. 211–228). New York: Academic Press.

Terry, R. D., & Katzman, R. (1983). Senile dementia Alzheimer's type. *Annals of Neurology, 14,* 497–506.

Weiner, M., Brok, A. J., & Snadowsky, A. M. (1987). *Work with the aged.* Stamford, CT: Appleton-Century-Crofts.

Weiner, M., Plutchik, R., & Rubino, J. (1991, August). *Coping styles as mediators of symptoms in the elderly.* Paper presented at the American Psychological Association Meeting. San Francisco, CA.

Wells, C. E. (1979). Pseudodementia. *American Journal of Psychiatry, 136,* 895–900.

Winokur, G. (1985). The validity of neurotic-reactive depression: New data and reappraisal. *Archives of General Psychiatry, 42,* 1116–1122.

6

Psychotherapeutic Approaches to the Depressed and Suicidal Older Person and Family

JOSEPH RICHMAN

This chapter discusses the place of psychotherapy in the treatment of suicidal states.

Suicidology, gerontology, and psychotherapy are all tied together in this endeavor because the suicide rate is highest in the elderly, and their psychological, social, and family experiences are intimately involved. I shall discuss some unfinished or insufficiently examined problems in the literature, especially as they relate to the treatment of the elderly person, and will present an overview of the general principles of psychotherapy with the suicidal elderly.

SUICIDE AS A FAMILY INHERITANCE

Because the family context is so important, a suicide by an adult parent or grandparent can result in an indelible stamp of self-destruction on others. Therefore, preventing elderly suicide can prevent youth suicides. Without treatment and prevention programs, the suicide of a member of the older generation can become a heritage to the younger.

For example, an elderly man, terminally ill with cancer, shot himself in the temple. Two months later, the newspapers reported on the suicide of his 16-year-old grandson, who also shot himself in the temple with the same gun. This tragedy occurred at the same time that Dr. Jack Kevorkian was helping Janet Adkins, his first victim, to commit suicide. However, the contrast between the publicity and wave of approval for the Kevorkian-assisted suicide and the lack of media attention to the preventable family tragedy of the grandfather and grandson is a sad commentary on our prevailing journalism values. I hope that a more balanced era is on the horizon.

ASSESSMENT

No matter what the treatment modality, the assessment must be as complete as possible. Bongar (1991) presents a comprehensive view of the legal as well as clinical ramifications of both the assessment and management of suicidal patients in various settings. Lettieri (1972) constructed different tables of risk factors for suicide, on the basis of age as well as sex, an interesting approach that deserves further investigation. The demographic, epidemiological, and clinical recognition signs that are associated with serious suicidal behavior in the elderly can be classified into 4 major areas as follows:

1. *Ego-weakening factors.* These include mental and physical illnesses, pain and other symptoms, alcoholism, and unremitting symptoms that do not respond to treatment. These contain a strong biological component, either in their etiology or in their effects.

2. *Social factors, as they impact on the vulnerable individual.* Suicide is associated with living alone, living in the inner city, having few or no friends, and possessing character traits that turn other people away. These are, of course, associated with isolation and alienation.

3. *Dynamic factors.* The most frequent have to do with loss, such as the death of a loved one. A history of suicidal behavior in the self and in family members is also included, in addition to current suicidal manifestations.

4. *Clinical factors and communications.* These include giving away prized possessions, and verbal and nonverbal expressions of depression, despair, hopelessness, and suicidal intent. Hints of a plan, such as storing up medication or buying a gun, are among such signs, as well as statements that the others will not have to worry about him or her for long.

These danger signs are contrasted with recovery factors, including present or potential strengths and resources of the suicidal individual, and the presence of actual or potential social supports and resources.

The preceding summary is incomplete because it pays too little attention to the context. Yet, the timing of a suicidal act is strongly determined by the situation. The role of the family is especially relevant; sometimes, the unit of treatment can fruitfully be considered the family itself (see Richman, 1993, for a detailed outline of the family assessment process).

Family factors include:

- *Severe disturbances in response to separation and loss.* The intensity of these reactions is based on early life experiences in the vulnerable individual, but also in other family members, often originating before the suicidal person was born. Two major results are an association of developmental and other necessary changes with unbearable separation anxiety, and an inability to grieve.

- *Roles and behavior disturbances.* These include double-binding and sadomasochistic relationships as well as difficulties in dealing with both positive affects (e.g., love and pleasure) and negative ones. Emotions are often primitive and poorly controlled; for example, intense rage combined with death wishes.

  The frequency of incest in the histories of suicidal people may be related to a complex of factors. Sexual drives impel children to relationships outside the family, which is a threat to families whose relationships are symbiotic and who cannot tolerate separation. Incest is related to an effort to keep family members from leaving. Success in other activities outside the family may also be viewed as a threat, including friendships developed by family members. They all pose a similar danger, the fear of loss.

- *A view of the outside world as a danger and a threat to the integrity of the family.* The result is a closed family system that may reject needed help during a suicidal state in one or more of its members.

- *Communication patterns within the family.* These include covert or indirect messages of helplessness, hopelessness, and stress in the family, which are blamed on the suicidal person, with covert or indirect messages concerning suicidal acts. Extreme secretiveness and denial round out what may be considered as a suicidogenic communication system within which the entire family is trapped.

- *The presence of a crisis that everyone perceives as intolerable.* This last crisis can be considered as the last straw, which is built on an accumulation of earlier but unresolved crises, combined with a compulsion to repeat and create new crises. Treatment of the suicidal must therefore be crisis oriented, and the therapist must be prepared for periodic crises.

Everyone working with the suicidal elderly should become familiar with the tables of individual, family, and other risk factors. They can serve as a valuable checklist of danger signs.

THE RISKS OF RISK ASSESSMENT

Every professional should also become aware that there may be risk factors in risk assessment and risk management such as diagnosis-precipitated suicides. Other more subtle factors are fears that treatment will undermine the structure and values of the family, as illustrated in the myth of exclusiveness, and the prevalence of false positives and false negatives in our assessment. The following sections discuss these risks.

Diagnosis-Precipitated Suicide

"Diagnosis-precipitated suicide" refers to suicidal reactions in vulnerable persons in response to the danger signs or diagnostic labels, whether true or false. One type is suicide precipitated by the examiner's or therapist's reporting of findings to the patient and family.

Consequently, assessment findings must be presented in a sensitive and empathic manner. Unknown to the therapist, suicide may be related to the irrational meaning that the patient and family attach to the diagnostic labels and treatment recommendations. Therefore, the meaning of the diagnosis or recommendations must be explored.

Suicidal reactions may also appear in the context of false or mistaken beliefs by suicidal patients and their families about their medical or psychiatric condition. Conwell (1991) presented the case of a 78-year-old man who shot himself in the chest, after finding blood in his stool, but miraculously survived. He had reacted to the mistaken belief that his colon cancer, which had been successfully treated with surgery, had returned. Tests disclosed that he did not have cancer or any other serious illness. He was relieved, happy to be alive, and grateful that he had not died.

Slaby (1992) described a 90-year-old woman with a conviction that she had AIDS. She suffered from an atypical monosymptomatic depression, which was successfully treated with ECT. That patient survived, but other patients were less fortunate. Clark (1992) studied suicides in the Chicago area and found that 15% of the elderly suicides were related to the patient's unfounded belief that he or she suffered from cancer or other major illnesses.

Suicide based on false diagnoses sometimes approach the delusional, as the example by Slaby illustrates. It is insufficiently recognized, however, that these are often shared beliefs or delusions, a kind of folie à deux, with a more deadly strength because of being shared.

For example, on September 20, 1992, the television program *A Current Affair* presented an account of a man who had helped his mother commit suicide because they believed she was suffering from cancer. It turned out that she did not have cancer. Nevertheless, her son proudly declared that he would do the same thing, were the situation to be repeated. That is a folie à deux, indeed, continuing even after the folly had led to death.

The play, *In My Defence,* based on the true story of Saskia Reeves—a 32-year-old woman who helped her mother, afflicted with Lou Gehrig's disease, commit suicide—described how she encouraged her mother to go through with the plan for assisted suicide when her mother began to have second thoughts.

My conclusion, derived from interviews with over 800 suicidal persons and families over the past 28 years, is that the vast majority of suicidal acts are assisted, in a passive or active manner, at a conscious or unconscious level.

Suicide and the "Myth of Exclusiveness"

To some patients and families, mental illness means the end of the road. They respond to such information with feelings of terror and despair, which in turn precipitates a suicidal act. Their fear may result in a covert and implacable resistance to treatment. One basis is the belief that any change in the suicidal person threatens the integrity or survival of the family system. The fear in such cases is compounded by the conviction that a close relationship, such as that between a therapist and patient, can take place only by destroying a previous close relationship, such as that between a mother and child.

The results may be fatal to the treatment. Suicidal patients may receive the covert and often unconscious message to fail. Rather than establishing a therapeutic alliance, the patient may resist, not respond to the treatment program, be it outpatient or hospitalization, and finally commit suicide.

Thus, failure in treatment may take place in the service of family loyalties. The suicide is then attributed to the unremitting nature of the person's symptoms, and the failure of the hospital or therapist to take sufficient precautions. The resulting litigation may serve to conceal the true situation. A family interview at the beginning of treatment will help decrease such fears and prevent many tragedies.

False Positives and False Negatives

A "false positive," refers to classifying someone as a high suicide risk, who spoils the statistics by not committing suicide. If errors must occur, I react with approval to such errors. Those who score high on the danger signs of suicide are usually unhappy, depressed, despairing people who feel hopeless. That they do not commit suicide is a tribute to their strengths, or the power of a caring support system, and most likely a combination of both. Even if they never commit suicide, they are in need of help.

"False negatives," not picking up the presence of a serious suicide risk when it is present, is a more serious problem. One recommendation is to see that the assessment includes the family and support systems; another is for the availability of supervisors and consultants who are experienced in suicidology and family interviewing; and a third is the availability of immediate treatment or crisis intervention. The risk of false negatives will be reduced when all health professionals receive adequate training and experience in recognizing suicidal risks.

THE ROADS TO SUICIDE PREVENTION

Some general principles in the treatment of elderly suicide apply to all the therapies. These include the need for a comprehensive assessment and a positive therapeutic relationship.

One of the enduring questions in therapy is fitting the treatment to the patient. That depends on a variety of factors, including the training and preferred style of the therapist, as well as the needs of the patient. It is desirable to determine when to choose one or another form of treatment. Individual therapy is effective in forming an intimate yet nonthreatening relationship. However, the patient does not exist in a family and social vacuum and neither does the treatment. It is essential that the family not perceive therapy as a threat to its integrity. For that purpose, family meetings are invaluable. The most effective approach, therefore, is a comprehensive one that may involve but not necessarily be limited to socially oriented interventions such as group or family therapy.

Group psychotherapy is recommended for the suicidal elderly because feelings of alienation are pervasive and often overwhelming. A sense of community helps the elderly cope with their many losses and feelings of loneliness and abandonment. The literature on group therapy with the suicidal uniformly finds that homogeneous groups, where all the patients are depressed and/or suicidal, are preferable to heterogeneous groups.

The volume on group psychotherapy for the elderly by MacLennan, Saul, and Weiner (1988) contains some valuable case history data (see also Richman, 1993, Chapter 6, pp. 134–144).

The group therapy sessions are lively and target symptom oriented, with much direct and open discussion of suicide and related topics. The group members discuss experiences with family members and others, as well as attitudes about hospitalization and other treatments such as ECT, with a degree of comfort and freedom much greater than in heterogeneous groups.

Family psychotherapy with the suicidal elderly is the treatment of choice because the family is involved not only in the tensions leading to a suicidal act but also in the eventual reduction of stress and suicidal reactions. Family therapy lessens separation and death anxiety. These reactions are based on early family experiences where change became associated with separation and loss, the breakdown of continuity, and a disruption of the family structure. When the threat of the repetition of these trauma is removed, there is often a leap forward in adjustment and development. Individual and group therapy can then take place with the implicit permission or approval of the family.

EARLY FAMILY EXPERIENCES AND SUICIDE

The family system is created through processes of introjection (Freud, 1917/1957), projection, and projective identification, and the splitting of good and bad, pleasant and unpleasant experiences among family members (Klein, 1975). One result of the splitting is that the outside world represents the bad and dangerous experiences, whereas the family represents the good. The closed family system arises out of such splitting.

And within the closed family, the splitting may continue, with different persons assigned good and bad roles. The setting is ripe, then, for the development of favoritism, blaming, and scapegoating.

Ross (1990), writing on the basis of painful personal experiences as the humiliated and scapegoated figure in her family, described the lessons she learned that enabled her to finally cope. "It is horrible to be or feel ostracized by your entire family," she wrote, and continued with sensitive understanding, "but that's the way of closed dysfunctional families" (Ross, 1990, p. 50). With the help of an adviser, she recognized that the family members had projected or transferred onto her whatever ugliness they had suffered in their own lives.

Ross possessed the wisdom and maturity to realize that understanding is only a beginning, but that understanding *"did* help me begin to forgive" (p. 51) wholeheartedly, not only intellectually. As she said, "I knew I had forgiven when I no longer felt . . . a desire to hurt back." Her story illustrates that understanding the role of the family in suicide is the major step toward healing and growth.

One other treatment resource that should not be neglected is the broad area of the creative art therapies, as Osgood (1985) recommended. For example, Mango (1992) described how art therapy served as a powerful instrument for tapping basic life-and-death issues in depth. Mango presented an extensive case history of a 71-year-old woman who was hospitalized on a psychiatric ward where she was seen in art psychotherapy. After 3 months, she was diagnosed with cancer of the liver and died within 3 weeks. Her drawings indicated that she unconsciously knew she was dying. Through the art therapy, she was expressing and coming to terms with her impending death.

Humor and storytelling are also among the creative arts. Many instances of humor occur during therapy with depressed and suicidal elderly patients (Richman, Brook, Carter, & Ross, 1991). Psychotherapy itself is a creative art. Like humor, psychotherapy recognizes the importance of surprise, good timing, and a positive relationship.

SPECIAL PROBLEMS

The Alleviation of Burdens

Virtually every suicidal person in my practice has stated that being a burden to others was a major reason for his or her suicidal intent. Being a burden has also been among the arguments in favor of "rational suicide" by the proponents of euthanasia. However, to be a burden is an interpersonal state, with strong family components.

An example was a 60-year-old woman who was treated for depression but did not improve. Her husband developed chest pains and her son symptoms of a stomach ulcer. "I am hurting everyone I love," said the woman and she committed suicide (Richman, 1986).

Unusual or uncharacteristic behavior by a relative is another communication of stress and burden. Derek Humphry (1986), for example, reported that he reacted to news that his first wife, Jean, had breast cancer, by going out and having sex with another woman. The therapeutic response is to alleviate the stress in the individual and the family system. During my assessment interviews, the feeling of burden in both the patient and others is covered and confronted at the beginning of treatment.

Death Wishes

Death wishes have been considered a major component of the suicidal act. Freud (1917/1957) regarded suicide as based on death wishes toward someone else turned against the self. Paul Federn, looking at the other side of the same coin, declared that no one kills himself unless his death is desired by someone else (in Maddison & Mackey, 1966). Death wishes by significant others have been reported frequently, and I have seen them regularly in my own practice (Rosenbaum & Richman, 1970).

Death wishes during both assessment and therapeutic interviews with suicidal patients are expressed most frequently by relatives. After seeing many patients and their families, I learned that the death wish could be the beginning of cure, when expressed during the therapy session. The meaning of the death wish is very different in a therapeutic situation than it is in the home. At some level, those involved in a family therapy session express rage and death wishes for a therapeutic intent: to make things better and as part of a healing process.

During the initial interviews, there is often an upsurge of intense emotional turmoil and rage. That is a good point for the therapist to intervene. I point out the positive aspects of their outbursts. They serve as an outlet for tensions and as an opportunity to express their feelings in a therapeutic setting. I then inquire into the most urgent danger signs. These include continuing depression and suicidal impulses, the exhaustion of the resources and coping abilities of the suicidal person and other family members, and the feelings of being a burden, as well as the presence of death wishes.

After further encouragement of the airing of conflicts and areas of tension, I relabel the expression of death wishes as a communication of complete exasperation and of not knowing how to respond or deal with the situation. This kind of reinterpretation or relabeling has been among the major measures for reducing tensions. Most often, what follows is a discussion of the most pressing situation leading to separation or death anxiety.

By pointing out that the expression of death wishes should not be taken literally, I am doing little more than placing their words or communications within a conventional social framework. The expression, "Drop dead," is stated frequently in anger but is not usually taken literally.

Humor makes a similar use of relabeling, for example, by switching from the metaphoric or emotional use of the expression, "Drop dead," to the literal. But when the death wish is taken literally in the context of severe stress and conflict, it is no joke. The solution is to recognize that the death wish is a metaphor and not a literal invitation to die. That therapeutic switch to restore the metaphoric meaning is accomplished through relabeling.

Such misunderstandings are a function of the relationship between the recipient and giver of the expression of death wishes. Most often, it is stated in family or other relationships where the people are involved in conflict. I recall a man in his 30s who went to his parents' house for Thanksgiving. During the meal, he had an argument with his parents, becoming very upset and excited. His father said to him, "You'll get an ulcer," meaning that he should calm down. However, the son took this statement as a curse that would come true, because he had dared to disagree with his father.

Death wishes are not only a communication of stress and conflict. They are also part of a pervasive preoccupation with death that is prevalent in suicidal persons. They also run through the long-term treatment of the suicidal elderly. Properly handled, an understanding of the preoccupation with death can be very therapeutic. Thoughts of death express an effort to cope with basic situations that have to do with life and caring relationships. They touch on people's need for each other, fears of abandonment, and the reassurance that the forces of love and loyalty will always be there.

The Misunderstandings and Neglect of Psychotherapy

Since 1965, I have devoted my professional career to treating suicide and other self-destructive behaviors and disasters. However, I have felt frustrated at the neglect of psychotherapy for the suicidal elderly. That is particularly true of family therapy. The professional literature, the news media, and the legal courts have all been replete with misunderstandings of the role of the family in the treatment, and prevention of destructive behaviors, as well as the role of the social network.

For example, Roazen (1969) studied the life and suicide of Victor Tausk, a promising young psychoanalyst whose paper on the influencing machine is still considered a major contribution to the understanding of paranoia. Tausk committed suicide in 1919.

Roazen studied Tausk and his suicide, and discovered that a troubled relationship with Sigmund Freud was a major determinant. His revelation of the role of important others in suicide paralleled my own early experiences in treating suicidal people in the 1960s. As a result, I moved from an understanding of suicide as an individual choice to suicide as intimately related to family and social network conflicts and tensions.

However, when Roazen found similar interpersonal dynamics, he took the traditional path of finding someone to blame. Rather than recognizing that the social aspects of suicide are found even among psychoanalysts, Roazen presented Freud's role in the death as a purely individual matter, the result of Freud's personal and professional failings.

Examples of such misunderstandings of the role of the family and social network in suicide are still pervasive. They are found in law, in literature, and most regrettably in psychology and psychiatry. They have been utilized by the proponents of "rational suicide" to neglect all forms of psychotherapy. Even professionals who have made important contributions to the understanding of the social context of suicide have demonstrated such misunderstandings.

For example, Kobler and Stotland (1964), a clinical and a social psychologist, studied an epidemic of suicides in a hospital that had had a long and successful treatment history, in which suicides were very rare. Changes in the administration, with the resulting development of a dysfunctional therapeutic setting, led to a sudden rash of suicides.

A social worker who described an interview with the mother of one of the patients who subsequently committed suicide in the hospital, wrote, "One interview was so full of death and morbidity in one form or another, including her statement that it would be easier to adjust to her son's death than to his mental illness, that I felt quite concerned about her and her ability to hold together."

I have heard such statements from the relatives of suicidal patients for over a quarter of a century. They express a severe state of tension and exhaustion in the family, as well as the patient. It is incumbent on the therapist to help relieve their stress. The expression of such feelings in therapy, especially when the patient is present, is a major step toward eventual cure. The therapist must know how to help the patient and family out of their morass.

Instead, however, Kobler and Stotland indignantly attributed the social worker's accurate remarks to her hostility toward the mother, and saw her only as the spokesperson for the negative attitude of the entire hospital staff toward the parents. These statements were published almost 30 years ago. Is it not time to correct such attitudes, which inhibit and prevent true therapeutic measures?

Nevertheless, such misunderstandings are still accepted uncritically, and therefore perpetuated. Over 20 years later, a 17-year-old go-go dancer in Florida killed herself. The government accused her mother of criminally driving her daughter to suicide, and a psychiatrist, Dr. Douglas Jacobs, testified for the prosecution that the mother had contributed to her daughter's death. The woman was found guilty and jailed.

The finding by lawyers and psychiatrists that the family was implicated in suicide should have been a call for encouraging research into family determinants and family therapy. Instead, the state blamed the mother, punished her, and as a result, no change or improvement in the treatment or prevention of suicide was needed. The only other outcome was that the television series *L.A. Law* presented a version of the Florida case, which continued the blaming of the mother, and ended in a burst of satisfaction that the mother was punished and justice was done.

Florida seems particularly vulnerable to respond with blame and punishment, rather than understanding. It continued the same pattern with the elderly involved in serious life crises in the case of Roswell Gilbert, a 75-year-old retiree who shot and killed his wife, a victim of Alzheimer's disease. Here was an example of the toll taken by dementia and other chronic disease on the family and caregivers. The message is for society to address itself to the problem. Instead, Florida found Mr. Gilbert guilty of murder and sentenced him to jail. Once again, nothing was learned and nothing was changed.

THE TREATABILITY OF
ELDERLY SUICIDE

There have been many papers on the conditions associated with elderly suicide, but few on its alleviation. Many elderly suicidal persons had seen a physician shortly before they killed themselves. It is recognized however, that doctors are woefully unprepared in their education and training for dealing with that population (Richman & Kahn, 1986).

Nevertheless, there is research evidence that physicians can play a significant role. In Gotland, Sweden (Rutz et al., 1989), general practitioners were educated in recognizing and treating depression. On that island, there was a significant reduction in the suicide rate, from 25 per 100,000 in 1982 to 7 per 100,000 in 1985. Such efforts are needed in the United States, too. The benefits are great, because preventing suicide not only saves lives but can prevent much additional grief and emotional disturbances among the survivors.

I have been particularly impressed by the therapeutic role of the family. Families contain forces of healing and growth that can be revived when the stresses around separation and discontinuity are reduced (Richman, 1993). Similar forces are present in group therapy (Reiss, 1968). A major task, therefore, in the treatment of suicide, is to replace deadly interactions with healing ones.

The same reasoning applies to suicide pacts and assisted suicides. Assisted living is probably more frequent and important than assisted suicide, but it is usually ignored. As Payne (1975) perceptively noted, a doctor's wish that a patient live has saved many lives. It goes without saying that the wish of the family and social network that a person live has saved even more lives. That is why there are not more suicides.

CONCLUSION

There are measures that society can take. One is the training of physicians and other health professionals. Another is outreach programs to identify and contact the suicidal elderly, in senior centers, adult homes, rehabilitation hospitals, and similar settings. More use can be made of crisis centers, telephone hot lines, and the medical and psychiatric emergency rooms of hospitals, not only for suicidal persons but for their relatives and other concerned persons.

An invaluable potential is to be found in the elderly themselves, with well elders helping the frail and sick. Thousands of older adults volunteer their services every day. Many of them can be trained as such helpers, and paid, in addition. It would be an investment well spent.

Education of the general public, including the use of the media, will be in the vanguard of suicide prevention in the 21st century. The best educators are those elderly who had been suicidal, overcome their self-destructive state, and went on to lead productive and meaningful lives. I can guarantee that they have inspiring stories to tell.

I urge the once suicidal or depressed elderly to appear on radio and television shows, to tell their stories. The suicidal who have recovered are the best role models to help others who are suicidal. Meanwhile, it behooves those of us in the health professions to devote more of our energies to the important and rewarding task of preventing and treating suicidal states in the elderly.

REFERENCES

Bongar, B. (1991). *The suicidal patient.* Washington, DC: American Psychological Association.

Clark, D. (1992, April 2). *Narcissistic crises of aging and elderly suicide.* Presidential address presented at the 25th annual conference of the American Association of Suicidology. Chicago, IL.

Conwell, Y. (1991, April 19). *A failed suicide.* Presented at the 24th annual conference of the American Association of Suicidology. Boston, MA.

Freud, S. (1957). Mourning and melancholia. In J. Strachey (Ed. and Trans.), *The Standard edition of the complete psychological works of Sigmund Freud* (Vol. 14, pp. 243–258). London: Hogarth Press. (Original work published 1917)

Humphry, D. (1986). *Jean's way.* New York: Harper & Row.

Klein, M. (1975). A contribution to the psychogenesis of manic-depressive states. In S. Lawrence (Ed.), *Love, guilt and reparation and other works, 1921–1945* (pp. 262–289). New York: Delacorte Press.

Kobler, A. L., & Stotland, E. (1964). *The end of hope.* New York: Free Press.

Lettieri, D. J. (1972). Suicide in the aging. Empirical prediction of suicidal risk among the aging. *Journal of Geriatric Psychiatry, 6,* 7–42.

MacLennan, B. W., Saul, S., & Weiner, M. B. (Eds.). (1988). *Group psychotherapies for the elderly* (American Group Psychotherapy Association Monograph 5). Madison, CT: International Universities Press.

Maddison, D., & Mackey, K. H. (1966). Suicide: The clinical problem. *British Journal of Psychiatry, 112,* 693–703.

Mango, C. (1992). Emma: Art therapy illustrating personal and universal images of loss. *Omega, 25*(4), 259–269.

Osgood, N. J. (1985). *Suicide in the elderly: A practitioner's guide to diagnosis and mental health intervention.* Rockville, MD: Aspen.

Payne, E. S. (1975). Depression and suicide. In J. G. Howells (Ed.), *Modern perspectives in the psychiatry of old age* (pp. 290–   ). New York: Brunner/Mazel.

Reiss, D. (1968). The suicide six: Observations on suicidal behavior and group function. *International Journal of Social Psychiatry, 14,* 201–212.

Richman, J. (1986). *Family therapy with suicidal persons* (pp. 134–144). New York: Springer.

Richman, J. (1993). *Preventing elderly suicide: Overcoming personal despair, professional neglect, and social bias.* New York: Springer.

Richman, J., Brook, A., Carter, B. F., & Ross, C. (1991). *Group suicide pre- and post vention, across the ages.* Presented at the 24th Annual Conference of the American Association of Suicidology, April 20, 1991. Boston, MA.

Richman, J., & Kahn, L. (1986, September 1–4). *Attitudes of physicians to physician's suicide.* Presented at the biannual conference of the International Association for Suicide Prevention. Vienna, Austria.

Roazen, P. (1969). *Brother animal. The story of Freud and Tausk.* New York: Knopf.

Rosenbaum, M. A., & Richman, J. (1970). Suicide: The role of hostility and death wishes from the family and significant others. *American Journal of Psychiatry, 126,* 128–131.

Ross, E. B. (1990). *After suicide: A ray of hope.* Iowa City, IA: Lynn Publications.

Rutz, W., Walinder, J., Eberhard, G., Holmberg, G., von Knorring, A-L, von Knorring, L., Wisted, B., & Aberg-Wisted, A. (1989). An educational program on depressive disorders for general practitioners on Gotland: Background and evaluation. *Acta Psychiatrica Scandinavica, 79,* 19–26.

Slaby, A. (1992, October 8). *The differential diagnosis and diagnostic specific management of suicidal behavior.* Paper presented at the Middletown Psychiatric Center, Middletown, NY.

7

Biological Treatment of Severe Late-Life Depression:
Pharmacotherapy and Electroconvulsive Therapy

DONALD P. HAY AND
LINDA K. HAY

Major depression is a severe illness, with prevalences varying from 1% to 2% in general populations to 12% in hospitals and nursing homes. Although depression is not more prevalent in older populations, when coupled with the multiplicity of physiological, psychological, and sociological stresses of aging, is a significant problem for the elderly (Allen & Blazer, 1991). Depressed mood, as a symptom that may or may not be associated with major depressive disorder, is the most common symptom in the elderly. Suicide is the most serious complication of depression, and the highest suicide rates occur in elderly white males (Allen & Blazer, 1991). Consequently, the treatment of depression in the elderly becomes an important issue for practitioners.

The diagnosis of depression involves consideration of clinical symptoms, psychiatric history, medication history, family history of affective disorder, and a thorough evaluation of any mitigating variables including physical health, environmental stresses, developmental crisis, support system, and coping mechanisms.

The physical workup is essential and consists of a thorough physical examination, a comprehensive health history, and a complete evaluation of all systems. Certain physical disorders and the medications used to treat them can produce symptoms of depression. Thus the primary step in evaluating and treating physical illness or eliminating certain medications may in itself resolve the patient's presenting psychiatric problems. The evaluation of physical health and current medications is also necessary before initiating any somatic treatment to prevent complications due to drug interactions or side effects.

The treatment of depression also includes the consideration of both psychiatric and physical problems, especially important in the elderly given the physical complications of aging, the numbers of medications used for the increased physical disorders, and the many vulnerabilities experienced by lessening social support, economic changes, and the developmental issues of aging. Treatment of major depression is often not considered because of the sometimes overwhelming physical concerns. Once the underlying physical causes of depression are resolved or ruled out, the treatment methods include psychotherapy, psychotropic medications, and electroconvulsive therapy (ECT).

In the more severe forms of major depression with melancholia, the somatic treatments are preferred, especially when suicidal potential is considered. Psychotherapy alone may be valuable in dysthymia and is especially important in the elderly because of the potentially deleterious side effects from antidepressant medications. Various modalities of psychotherapy are employed with older patients with much the same results as with younger patients. Psychotherapy may also enhance somatic treatments and is a recommended adjunct to other treatment modalities.

In discussing the use of chemotherapy and ECT in older patients and especially in those with suicidal potential, several issues emerge. Though commonalities with younger patients exist, the selection of antidepressant medication must be carefully weighed in terms of potential side effects and their interaction with the multiple medications that most older individuals are taking. In addition, dosage, frequency of complications, duration of treatment, compliance, and response rates are important variables when treating the elderly.

Failure to treat and undertreatment are often apparent with elderly depressed patients. Health care providers and family members may be uninformed as to the treatability of depression in the elderly because the misconception persists that depression is a "normal" response to age.

Undertreatment occurs when health care providers are not familiar with the benefits and limitations of psychiatric medications. Frequently, an antidepressant is prescribed for an elderly patient at a minimal, sub-therapeutic dose, and the patient is not evaluated as often as necessary to monitor the response and to increase the dose as warranted.

The use of ECT also involves special considerations in elderly patients. These include the pre-ECT medical workup, adequate informed consent, and various procedural issues such as dosage, choice of stimulating device (type of electrical waveform), electrode placement, frequency of treatment, and use of maintenance ECT.

PHARMACOTHERAPY

Pharmacology of Aging

An emerging science differentiates the psychopharmacology of older adults from that of younger adults. Age-related changes of the body and the central nervous system may result in the elderly having responses to psychiatric medications that differ from those of younger adults.

Changes in pharmacokinetics or alteration in drug biotransformation and disposition represent one type of age-related difference. There are several significant differences noted in older individuals such as decreased absorption, as well as altered metabolism, distribution, and excretion of medications.

Absorption of medications occurs in the gastrointestinal tract by diffusion. There is evidence of decreased rate of absorption of lipid soluble drugs with age, but in general, most psychotropic medications are totally absorbed by the elderly (Israili & Wenger, 1981).

The liver is the main area for metabolism of psychotropic drugs that are lipid-soluble. Age-associated hepatic changes may cause a slowing of drug metabolism (Greenblatt & Shader, 1982). This in turn contributes to higher blood levels of some psychotropic medications such as benzodiazepines and tricyclics. Blood levels, however, are also affected by distribution and excretion.

Distribution of drugs occurs in fat tissue, body water, and plasma proteins. Since most psychotropic drugs, with the exception of lithium, are lipid soluble and distributed in fat tissue, and body fat increases with age, the volume of distribution of psychotropic drugs in the elderly is increased (Hollister, 1981). Aging also affects plasma proteins that may increase concentrations of plasma lithium and other hydrophilic drug metabolites.

The elimination of psychotropic drugs occur by way of the kidneys. A decrease in the glomerular filtration rate that occurs in older adults may increase the accumulation of metabolites in older individuals (Young et al., 1984).

It is important to consider increased plasma concentration of drugs in the elderly caused by changes in absorption, metabolism, distribution, and elimination as a result of steady-state concentrations. Half-life is the amount of time necessary to eliminate half the amount of a drug. Steady-state is achieved when the amount of a drug entering the plasma equals the amount being eliminated. Since the half-life of most drugs is increased in the elderly, it takes longer to achieve the steady-state of plasma concentration. This has implications in the monitoring of the administration of psychotropic medications in the elderly in terms of the therapeutic response time.

In addition to changes of aging, pharmacokinetics are also affected by physical illnesses, often more prevalent in the elderly, and can also lead to decreased absorption and diminished renal functioning. The drugs and diets used to manage physical illnesses can interact at a pharmacokinetic level as well as produce changes in concentration in both psychotropic and nonpsychotropic drugs.

Pharmacodynamic changes, the alteration in central nervous system response to drugs, also occur in older individuals. Aging decreases the number of neurons, decreases activity of synthetic enzymes, decreases neurotransmitter concentration, possibly decreases the binding of presynaptic neurotransmitter receptors, increases monamine oxidase, decreases the density of neurotransmitters in the postsynaptic receptor, and decreases the sensitivity and increases the density of drug receptors (Young et al., 1984).

The implications of the effects of aging on pharmacodynamics are complicated by the different neurotransmitter systems involved with different drugs, the interaction of these various systems and the effect of chronic administration. It may be postulated, however, that decreased dopamine function, for example, may lead to the increase of the incidence of extrapyramidal side effects in patients taking neuroleptics. In addition, the decrease in central nervous system acetylcholine when combined with the administration of tricyclic antidepressants that affect acetylcholine function may lead to increased confusion, disorientation, and memory loss (Salzman, 1984). Ultimately, empirical studies are called for to establish better clinical guidelines related to the increased sensitivity to psychotropic medication in the elderly.

Certain disorders of the central nervous system can also change the effects of drugs. Parkinson's disease, cerebrovascular disease, and primary degenerative dementia have been known to disrupt neurotransmitter systems. The implication is that these central nervous system disorders may produce an increased sensitivity to psychotropic medications and their side effects such as motor dysfunction and anticholinergic effects.

In addition to differences in drug responses and metabolism between younger and older patients, there are age-related problems in the quantity of drugs prescribed as well as compliance. Older individuals frequently take several types of medication at once. This increases the risk of drug interactions that could lead to toxic side effects or inhibit the therapeutic effect of any medication. The quantity of drugs prescribed for an older individual contributes to lack of compliance in that multiple drug regimens are complicated and difficult to complete.

The optimal therapeutic effect of an antidepressant is positively correlated to the plasma level. The optimal plasma level for cyclic antidepressants in the elderly has not been determined. It is important to use lower doses than in younger individuals, however, due to the physical changes of aging. For an initial dose of any antidepressant, 10 to 25 mg of most typical tricyclic antidepressants would be safe with an increase of 10 or 25 mg every 2 to 4 days until a clinical response is achieved. If there is no clinical response, plasma levels may be checked before switching to another antidepressant.

Drug Classes

Tricyclic antidepressants (TCAs) and the newer heterocyclic antidepressants are the main treatment choice for depression. Since there is no clinical evidence that one cyclic antidepressant is best, the choice of antidepressant is usually made on the basis of consideration of the pharmacokinetic factors, side effects, the patient's physical health, and history of prior drug response. The cyclic antidepressants, therefore, can be discussed from the perspective of groupings including tertiary versus secondary amine metabolites and serotonin reuptake blockers, as well as the side effect profiles of sedation, cardiotoxicity, orthostatic hypotension, anticholinergic effects, and impaired memory function (see Table 7–1).

Of the TCAs, the tertiary amines such as imipramine, amitriptyline, and doxepin are likely to be more concentrated than the secondary amines such as desipramine (Norpramin) and nortryptyline (Pamelor), which require one less phase of hepatic metabolism. The

TABLE 7–1
Antidepressants: Side Effects

Drug	Anticholingeric	Sedation	Hypotension	Cardiotoxicity
Tertiary amines				
Imipramine	+ +-+ + +	+	+ +	+ +
Doxepin	+ + +	+ +-+ + +	+ +	+ +
Amitryptyline	+ + + +	+ + +	+ +	+ + +
Trimipramine	+ + +	+ + +	+ +	+ + +
Secondary amines				
Desipramine	+	+	+-+ +	+
Nortriptyline	+ +	+	+	+
Amoxapine	+ +	+	+ +	+ +
Protriptyline	+ + +	+	+ +	+ +
Maprotiline	+ +	+ +-+ + +	+ +	+
Atypical				
Trazodone	+	+ +	+ +	+-+ +
Fluoxetine	+	-	+	+
Buproprion	+	-	+	+
Sertraline	+	-	+	+

+ mild
+ + moderate
+ + + strong
+ + + + very strong
- activating

References: Salzman, 1984; Rickels & Schweizer, 1990.

lower concentrations of the secondary amines produce less side effects such as orthostatic hypotension and sedation compared with the tertiary amines (Salzman, 1984).

Clinical response to antidepressants is dose related, and low doses of some antidepressants of any type may be very helpful without having the toxic side effects that might occur at higher doses. Some older individuals may require the same dose as younger individuals to achieve a therapeutic effect thus increasing the potential for cardiac toxicity and prolonged electrical conduction that could lead to heart block and ventricular arrhythmias. Electrocardiograms establishing normal conduction may be used to monitor the increase of a cyclic antidepressant (Salzman, 1984).

The serotonin reuptake blockers such as trazodone, fluoxetine, and sertraline, as well as buproprion, are comparable to the secondary amines in terms of low anticholinergic properties. Trazodone is especially helpful for the geriatric patient who requires sedation, and it has been used for the treatment of agitation as an alternative or adjunct to neuroleptics and/or benzodiazepines (Simpson & Foster, 1986). This may have widespread implications because the extensive use of neuroleptics has the potential for extrapyramidal side effects and tardive dyskinesia, and benzodiazepines have the potential for falls. Fluoxetine is useful in treating older patients who require a more activating antidepressant.

Even though the use of the cyclic antidepressants is relatively safe, there are several concerns. There may be a potential for cardiotoxicity and a greater sensitivity to side effects such as impaired memory function related to anticholinergic qualities of antidepressants. Memory impairment is especially troublesome for aging patients as this may be mistaken for dementia.

Buspirone, another serotonergic reuptake blocker, may be helpful in combination with an antidepressant and an intermediate half-life benzodiazepine for the agitated depressed patient. As the patient's acute symptoms lessen, the dose of buspirone can be increased while the dose of benzodiazepine is reduced.

Monoamine oxidase inhibitors (MAOIs) are sometimes very effective in treating major depressive illness in the elderly. The MAOIs may be an excellent choice of treatment for the patient who has not been helped by the cyclic antidepressants. No specific MAOI has ever been shown to be superior over the others, and the choice is usually based on clinical preference (Salzman, 1984).

Lithium is used to treat bipolar affective disorder in the elderly much the same as in younger patients. However, the clinician must be cautious given the increased potential for toxicity as well as potential for effect on renal, cardiac, and thyroid function; pretreatment evaluation of these systems is essential. When physical illness exists, serious toxicity may result.

Neuroleptics are used for the management of psychotic symptoms associated with depressive disorders, and antianxiety agents may be used to treat the symptoms of anxiety and agitation that may occur. The administration of each of these drug classes requires knowledge of the differences encountered when treating older patients. In most cases, the doses of these drugs must be reduced in older patients (see Table 7–2).

Behavioral symptoms of agitation and anxiety in the elderly including those with dementia frequently pose difficult treatment obstacles. The cyclic antidepressants with sedating side effects are often used instead of neuroleptics or antianxiety agents in the elderly. Because their side

TABLE 7–2
Geriatric Dosages

Generic Name	Trade Name	Approximate Daily Dosage in Milligrams
Cyclic Antidepressants		
Amitryptyline	Elavil	10–75
Amoxapine	Asendin	25–300
Desipramine	Norpramin	10–75
Doxepin	Sinequan	10–75
Imipramine	Tofranil	10–75
Maprotiline	Ludiomil	10–75
Nortriptyline	Pamelor	10–50
Protriptyline	Vivactil	5–20
Trazodone	Desyrel	25–400
Trimipramine	Surmontil	10–75
Atypical Antidepressants		
Fluoxetine	Prozac	10
Buproprion	Wellbutrin	75–200
Sertraline	Zoloft	25–100
MAO Inhibitors		
Isocarboxazid	Marplan	10–30
Phenelzine	Nardil	15–45
Tranylcypromine	Parnate	10–30

References: Salzman, 1984; Rickels & Schweizer, 1990.

effect profile may be relatively safer than the antipsychotics (potential for extra pyramidal side effects and tardive dyskinesia) and benzodiazepines (potential for excessive sedation or falls when used long term), the use of an antidepressant with low anticholinergic side effects such as trazodone for anxiety, agitation, and insomnia in the elderly, especially those with "organic affective syndrome," may be a prudent approach.

ELECTROCONVULSIVE THERAPY

Electroconvulsive therapy (ECT), although often misunderstood, continues to be an extremely effective treatment for depression as well as for bipolar disorder and schizoaffective disorders, especially in the elderly. Frequently, elderly patients are not able to tolerate the side effects of antidepressant medications either alone or in combination with the other medications they are taking, as well as the additive effect of the physical complications of diseases in other organ systems. ECT is a safe and effective alternative to medication for older depressed patients who may be agitated, withdrawn, or delusional (Hay, 1991).

The combination of the low risk of side effects from ECT and the findings that depression itself can increase mortality rates in elderly medically ill patients with severe physical illness make it imperative to recognize ECT as an essential treatment. It has been reported that older patients respond as well as if not better than younger patients to ECT (Stromgren, 1973).

The primary concern with the use of ECT in the elderly then, is not its efficacy or speed of onset of action (much greater than medication), but that of evaluating the patient in terms of the increased number of medical problems and the subsequent medication profile.

Indications for ECT

Many studies have demonstrated ECT to be an effective treatment for depressive illness, mania, and acute schizophrenic episodes with an affective component (Abrams, 1988; Endler & Persad, 1988). The use of ECT for situational sadness, unhappiness, dysthymic disorder, personality disorder, or characterological disorder is not considered to be appropriate. ECT has been considered appropriate for some medical disorders including catatonia, intractable seizure disorder, neuroleptic malignant syndrome, Parkinson's disease, and some situations of tardive dyskinesia (Hay, 1991; Hay & Hay, 1990).

The indications for the use of ECT in the elderly is basically the same as for its use in younger individuals. ECT is frequently found to be more effective and associated with less risk than psychopharmacological treatments in older individuals. In the elderly, ECT is used to treat major depressive disorder more frequently than any other mental illness in the *Diagnostic and Statistical Manual of Mental Disorders* (DSM-III-R, DSM-IV; American Psychiatric Association, 1994).

Pseudodementia has been described as a syndrome in the elderly with symptoms of disorientation and impaired cognition that are associated with depression and often misdiagnosed as dementia. Individuals with this presentation often respond well to ECT if they are unable to tolerate the side effects of the antidepressants. In patients with genuine dementia, such as Alzheimer's disease, with concomitant symptoms of depression and agitation, and as seen frequently in organic affective syndrome,

ECT may be effective in modifying mood and is not associated with increasing the dementia.

There are specific predictors of good outcome of ECT in the depressed elderly. These include major mood disorder, guilt, psychomotor retardation, and coexistent symptoms of agitation and anxiety (Fraser & Glass, 1980). In addition, nonresponsiveness to psychotropic medication, serious suicidal risk, refusal to eat or drink, insomnia, history of better response to ECT than to other treatment, and delusions are all indications for the choice of ECT in the elderly. In fact, delusional depression, which is difficult to treat in the elderly patient because of the greater potential for side effects before achieving adequate levels of neuroleptic and antidepressant, may best be treated by proceeding directly to ECT.

Contraindications

There are few absolute contraindications for ECT in the elderly and even these must be balanced against the risk of the continuing depression and other treatment modalities. To lessen the risk of ECT with concurrent medical illnesses such as recent myocardial infarction, congestive heart failure, conduction abnormalities, hypertension, and impaired pulmonary function, specific medical measures prior to ECT may be instituted with the aid of a consulting specialist. Increased intracranial pressure has usually been considered an absolute contraindication to ECT. However, each situation must be viewed as a unique event, and the risk-benefit ratio of *giving the treatment* must be weighed against the risk-benefit ratio of *not giving the treatment.*

Adverse Effects

The mortality rate for ECT is essentially the same as from anesthesia alone, approximately three or four deaths per 100,000 treatments or one death per 10,000 patients treated (Abrams, 1988; Fink, 1979). The most frequently reported cause of death associated with ECT has been cardiovascular complication.

The occurrence of confusion and/or memory loss after ECT is variable depending on electrode placement, type of stimulus, length of seizure activity, number of previous treatments, and spacing between treatments. This is more of an issue for the elderly who are more vulnerable to the multiple systemic problems associated with cognition impairment as well as the negative effects of depression alone on memory and concentration.

Unilateral electrode placement and brief-pulse stimulation have been associated with less postictal confusion and earlier reorientation. Most elderly patients treated with nondominant hemisphere and brief-pulse stimulus ECT exhibit little if any worsening of cognition or memory loss, especially of any lasting consequence. Conversely, it is frequently dramatic and heartening to see significant *improvement* in cognition and memory in patients in whom depressive illness had exerted a severe sensorium dysfunction.

Procedure

Informed consent is an essential and often difficult component in the process of ECT with the elderly. If the patient cannot consent to treatment, in most states the procedure cannot be initiated without a court order. In some cases, the patient cannot provide adequate consent as a direct consequence of the symptoms of severe depression including delusional ideation or impaired cognition. Family members are a great source in the educational process of informed consent and are utilized more frequently with older adults. In some cases, it is necessary to obtain a court order if delaying the treatment may be life threatening.

Pretreatment assessment should be especially thorough for the older adult. This includes a biochemistry screening panel, thyroid function tests, urinalysis, electrocardiogram, chest X ray, and physical exam with adequate neurological assessment. Complete spinal X rays may be necessary more often in older individuals given the more frequent occurrence of fractures, osteoporosis, or other spinal degeneration. Careful evaluation of the dentition of the elderly patient is essential. Full and partial dental plates should be removed prior to ECT to prevent damage, and the use of a semicircular rubber bite block is recommended so as to distribute pressure associated with the clenching of the masseter muscle.

Older patients frequently have a higher seizure threshold, and the seizure duration decreases with age such that elderly patients may require higher energy levels (Fogel, 1988). The choice of laterality of electrode placement in the elderly is complicated by the competing variables of known increased clinical efficacy of bilateral ECT but the greater potential in the elderly for memory loss or confusion with bilateral treatments. For this reason, at some centers right unilateral ECT is used initially in the elderly; but if it is insufficiently effective, it is replaced with bilateral.

Treatment frequency varies, with three times a week as the most usual pattern in the United States (twice a week in the United Kingdom). The total number of ECT treatments in a series is usually 6 to 9 for the elderly, although 12 or more may be necessary for some. The treatment continues until the patient is symptom free, unless confusion or persistent memory loss supervene.

Premedication with an anticholinergic agent such as atropine or glycopyrrolate is used to block the vagal effects on the heart. Glycopyrrolate, an agent that does not enter the central nervous system may be preferred in the elderly as it is less likely to promote postictal confusion and cardiac arrhythmias (Abrams, 1988).

The choice of anesthetic in the elderly is usually methohexital as it reportedly induces fewer cardiac arrhythmias than thiopental (Abrams, 1988). There is also a shorter sleep time and less confusion associated with methohexital.

In elderly patients, there is a greater potential for fractures, and a slightly higher dose of muscle relaxant (succinylcholine) may be necessary. It is also essential to wait for the cessation of the succinylcholine-induced faciculations in the gastrocnemius muscle and toes before proceeding with the ECT stimulation. Circulation in the elderly is slower and administering the ECT stimulus prior to complete paralysis could put a patient at greater risk for fractures. Use of a handheld nerve stimulator to check for total muscular relaxation is very helpful.

It is extremely important to cuff-off a lower extremity that is not compromised vascularly to observe for the presence of an induced seizure. Missed seizures may be misconstrued as ineffective treatment. If a seizure is not induced after the first impulse, another impulse may be administered immediately at a higher dosage setting so that the patient will not have to undergo anesthesia and its potential risks any more than is necessary.

Oxygenation with 100% oxygen is essential when treating the elderly with ECT as well as for younger adults due to the increase in cerebral oxygen requirements. This tends to decrease the side effects of memory loss and cardiac arrhythmias.

The treating psychiatrist is wise to alert the rest of the treatment team, including the anesthesiologist, recovery room nurses, and unit nurses, to the special needs of the elderly. This will ensure that the special measures used to promote a safe outcome will be understood and initiated by the entire treatment team, some of whom may not be familiar with the different techniques used with older patients.

Maintenance ECT

An important clinical issue is the avoidance of relapse. A usual post ECT regimen includes placing the patient on antidepressant medication or lithium. Maintenance ECT is recommended for patients who have shown a prior positive response to ECT and have had a relapse within 6 months of completion of an initial ECT series despite adequate dose of antidepressant. More recent information indicates that the 15% to 20% relapse rate in patients post ECT and on maintenance pharmacotherapy may in fact be greater, approaching 50% (Sackheim et al., 1990). This may lead to offering to patients the option of *continuation* ECT with a gradual tapering schedule after the main series is completed.

Maintenance ECT is initiated approximately one week after the series is completed. Thereafter, the interval between treatments is increased such that the patient receives four to six treatments over a 6-month period. Any return of symptoms requires a shortening of the interval.

CONCLUSION

Both chemotherapy and ECT have essential roles in the treatment of major depression in the elderly. There are several considerations that modify these treatments to meet the needs of the older adult. With careful administration and awareness of the physiological changes of aging, antidepressant medication and ECT can be lifesaving interventions.

REFERENCES

Abrams, R. (1988). *Electroconvulsive therapy.* New York: Oxford University Press.

Allen, A., & Blazer, D. G. (1991). Mood disorders. In J. Sadovoy, L. W. Lazarus, & L. F. Jarvik (Eds.), *Comprehensive review of geriatric psychiatry* (pp. 337–351). Washington, DC: American Psychiatric Press.

American Psychiatric Association. (1987, 1994). *The diagnostic and statistical manual of mental disorders* (3rd. ed. rev., 4th ed.). Washington, DC: Author.

American Psychiatric Association. (1990). The practice of electroconvulsive therapy: Recommendations for treatment, training, and privileging. Washington, DC: Author.

Endler, N. S., & Persad, E. (1988). *Electroconvulsive therapy: The myths and the realities.* Toronto: Hans Huber.

Fink, M. (1979). *Convulsive therapy: Theory and practice.* New York: Raven Press.

Fogel, B. (1988). Electroconvulsive therapy in the elderly: A clinical research agenda. *International Journal of Geriatric Psychiatry, 3,* 181–190.

Fraser, R., & Glass, I. B. (1980). Unilateral and bilateral ECT in elderly patients. *Acta Psychiatrica Scandinavica, 62,* 13–31.

Greenblatt, D. J., & Shader, R. J. (1982). Benzodiazepine kinetics in the elderly. In E. Usdin (Ed.), *Clinical Pharmacology in Psychiatry* (pp. 174–181), New York: Elsevier.

Hay, D. (1991). Electroconvulsive therapy. In J. Sadavoy, J. W. Lazarus, & L. F. Jarvik (Eds.), *Comprehensive review of geriatric psychiatry* (pp. 469–485). Washington, DC: American Psychiatric Press.

Hay, D., & Hay, L. (1990). The role of ECT in the treatment of depression. In C. D. McCann & N. S. Endler (Eds.), *Depression: New directions in theory, research, and practice* (pp. 255–272). Toronto: Wall & Emerson.

Hollister, L. E. (1981). General principles of treating the elderly with drugs. In L. Jarvik, D. J. Greenblatt, & D. Harmon (Eds.), *Clinical pharmacology and the aging patient* (pp. 1–9). New York: Raven Press.

Israili, Z. H., & Wenger, J. (1981). Aging, gastrointestinal disease, and response to drugs. In L. Jarvik, D. J. Greenblatt, & D. Harman (Eds.), *Clinical pharmacology and the aging patient* (pp. 131–155). New York: Raven Press.

Rickels, K., & Schweizer, E. (1990). Clinical overview of serotonin reuptake inhibitors. *Journal of Clinical Psychiatry, 51,* 9–12.

Sackheim, H. A., Prudic, J., Devanand, D. P., Decina, P., Kerr, B., & Malitz, S. (1990). The impact of medication resistance and continuation pharmacotherapy on relapse following response to ECT in major depression. *Journal of Clinical Psychopharmacology, 10,* 96–104.

Salzman, C. (1984). *Clinical geriatric psychopharmacology.* New York: Mc-Graw-Hill.

Simpson, D. M., & Foster, D. (1986). Improvement in organically disturbed behavior with trazodone treatment. *Journal of Clinical Psychiatry, 47,* 191–193.

Stromgren, L. S. (1973). Unilateral versus bilateral electroconvulsive therapy: Investigations into the therapeutic effect in endogenous depression. *Acta Psychiatrica Scandinavica, 240,* 8–65.

Welch, C. (1988). *Electroconvulsive therapy* (Manual of psychiatric treatment). Washington, DC: American Psychiatric Association.

Young, R. C., Alexopoulos, G. S., Shamoian, C. A., Manley, M. W., Dhar, A. K., & Kutt, H. (1984). Plasma 10-hydroxynortriptyline in elderly depressed patients. *Clinical Pharmacology and Therapy, 35,* 540–544.

8

A Brief Antidepressant
Prescribing Guide
for the Generalist

GARY J. KENNEDY

The discovery of antidepressant medications has progressed from empiricism to theory-driven "designer drugs" that manipulate mechanisms of monoamine neurotransmission (Richelson, 1994). This had led to a virtual golden age of psychotropic choices that can leave the generalist provider bewildered by the expanding array of highly touted pharmaceuticals (Ereshefsky, Overman, & Karp, 1995; Pollock, 1994). Here we offer a prescribing guide with preferences and precautions tailored to the generalist.

Before a clinician prescribes, it is necessary to consider the patient's risk of suicide and potential toxicity of a given agent. The selective serotonergic reuptake inhibitors are relatively free of life-threatening side effects (Crewe, Lennard, Tucker, Woods, & Haddock, 1992; Druckenbrod & Mulsant, 1994). However polypharmacy can complicate and endanger even the most cautious approach (Brymer & Winograd, 1992). As the number of medications increases, the risk of adverse reactions or interaction multiplies. Human factors must also be taken into account.

133

The more complex the regimen, the greater the error rate in even the most compliant, compulsive patient. Social isolation means the patient may not have a concerned party to reinforce the regimen, pick up a forgotten dose or be vigilant for dangerous side effects. Costs of the most recently introduced agents are substantially greater than the drugs that have become available generically. Physical illness, frailty, and cognitive impairment further argue for conservatism.

However, the clinical indications for the use of antidepressants have expanded in recent years to include anxiety disorders, sleep disturbance, and chronic pain syndromes as well as depressive disorders.

With the introduction of medications without life-threatening side effects (Hyttel, 1994) and the focus on the need to prevent recurrence as well as induce remission, controversy has arisen regarding the duration of antidepressant treatment. For recurrent depression, treatment may well need to be lifelong with the risks of undesirable side effects being overshadowed by the potentially permanent loss of capacity occasioned by recurrence. Risk can be minimized but not eliminated.

Minimizing the risk of adverse reactions depends in part on recognition of pharmacokinetics and dynamics of antidepressant medications. Of the pharmacokinetic properties of antidepressants, absorption is the least important consideration in regard to advanced age, followed by excretion, distribution, and metabolism in order of importance. Regarding pharmacodynamics, it is important to be aware of the dose-response relationship. Highly selective agents may become less so as the dose is increased. Both efficacy and adverse reactions are more likely as well. For agents with hypotensive, arrhythmic, and amnestic side effects, risk of an adverse reaction may be negligible at low doses (Pollock, Perel, Paradis, Fasicka, & Reynolds, 1994). Interindividual variability increases with age. An adequate trial of medication may take longer for an older adult than a younger person, but some seniors will tolerate and require the amount of medication appropriate for a person half their age.

Patients should be made aware of the latency of effect on mood. With the more sedative antidepressants, however, beneficial effects on sleep disturbance and anxiety may be realized within the first days of treatment (Lawlor, 1990). Similarly, most adverse reactions will occur in the early stage of treatment. Thus it is essential to counsel patients as to which side effects should be seen as tolerable and which are intolerable. Dry mouth, constipation, vivid dreams, temporary increase in anxiety, and tremor are not cause for alarm. Lowered blood pressure, syncope, and cardiac arrhythmia are warning signs of potentially dangerous adverse reactions.

Table 8–1 is a list of agents from each of the major antidepressant classes, and Table 8–2 is a more complete guide to the more commonly used and most recently introduced antidepressants.

TABLE 8–1

Representative Choices from the Major Classes of Antidepressants

Drug	Dosage	Side Effects
Nortriptyline *(Pamelor)*	Start at 10 mg, stop at 150 (hs), therapeutic window	Low amnesia and hypotension risk but sedative and pro-arrhythmic at high dose
Sertraline *(Zoloft)*	Start at 50 mg, stop at 200 mg (BID!)	No risk of amnesia, arrhythmia, not hypotensive but not sedative
		Weight loss, nausea are principal risks
Trazodone *(Desyrel)*	Start at 50 mg, stop at 300 (hs)	No risk of amnesia or arrhythmia, but hypotensive and quite sedative
Maprotiline *(Ludiomil)*	Start at 25 mg, stop at 225 mg (hs)	Low amnesia and arrhythmia risk but sedative and hypotensive
Bupropion *(Wellbutrin)*	Start at 50 mg, stop at 300 mg (BID!/TID!)	No risk of amnesia, arrhythmia, not hypotensive but not sedative
		Seizures, weight loss are principal risks
Tranlycypromine *(Parnate)*	Start at 10 mg, stop at 60 mg (BID!/TID!)	No risk of amnesia or arrhythmia
		Hypotensive but not sedative
		Dangerous interactions with food and drugs
Methylphenidate *(Ritalin)*	Start at 5 mg, stop at 60 (BID! before meals)	No risk of amnesia, hypotension, sedation
		Arrhythmogenic, anxiogenic, weight loss

TABLE 8-2

Identification, Prescription, and Precautions for Antidepressant Medications in Old Age

Generic Name	Trade Name	Initial Dose	Final Dose	Amnesia, Arrhythmia Potential	Hypotensive Potential	Sedative Potential	Precautions	Advantages
Tricyclic (TCAs)								
Amitriptyline	Elavil, Endep	10–25	50–300	High	High	High	In older or physically ill patients	Sedative
Nortriptyline	Pamelor Aventyl	10–25	50–100	Moderate	Moderate	Moderate	Lower final dose	Therapeutic window 50–150 ng/ml
Imipramine	Tofranil	10–25	50–300	Moderate	High	Moderate	In older or physically ill patients	Ther. level 150–250 ng/ml
Desipramine	Norpramin	10–25	100–200	Low	Moderate	Low	Purely noradrenergic	Ther. level 125–300 ng/ml; Stimulant
Doxepin	Sinequan Adapin	10–25	50–300	Moderate	Moderate	High	In older or physically ill patients	Sedative
Tetracyclic								
Amoxapine	Asendin	25	75–300	Moderate	Moderate	High	Tardive dyskinesia, dystonia	Neuroleptic anti-depressant
Maprotiline	Ludiomil	25	75–150	Moderate	Moderate	High	Seizures	
Selective Serotonergic Reuptake Inhibitors (SSRIs)								
Fluoxetine	Prozac	10–20	20–60	Low	Low	Low	Prolonged $T_{1/2}$[a]. nausea, tremor, insomnia	Side effects not life threatening
Sertraline	Zoloft	25–50	100–200	Low	Low	Low	Nausea, tremor, insomnia	(see Prozac)
Paroxetine	Paxil	10–20	20–40	Low	Low	Low	Nausea, tremor, insomnia	(see Prozac)
Venlafaxine	Effexor	25–50	75–225	Low	Low	Low	Hypertensive, anorexic	SSRI & SNRI[b]

Monoamine Oxidase Inhibitors (MAOIs)

Phenelzine	*Nardil*	15–30	45–60	Low	Moderate	Low	Life-threatening diet & drug interactions, prolonged $T\frac{1}{2}$[a]	When depression resists TCA/SSRI
Tranylcypromine	*Parnate*	10–20	30–60	Low	Moderate	Low	Life-threatening diet & drug interactions	When depression resists TCA/SSRI, Stimulant, short $T\frac{1}{2}$[a]
Others								
Bupropion	*Wellbutrin*	50–75	200–300	Low	Low	Low	Purely noradrenergic, seizures, dose should be divided	Anxiolytic
Nefazadone	*Serzone*	50	200–400	Low	Moderate	Moderate	Dry mouth; divide the dose	Sedative SSRI
Trazodone	*Desyrel*	25–50	100–400	Low	High	High	Very sedative, no partial response	For sleep disturbance
Stimulants								
Methylphenidate	*Ritalin*	5–10	20–60	Low	Low	Low	Anorexia, insomnia, for A.M. only	Quick results, for the frail and apathetic

[a] $T\frac{1}{2}$ = half-life.
[b] SNRI = selective noradrenergic reuptake inhibitor.

137

REFERENCES

Brymer, C., & Winograd, C. (1992). Fluoxetine in elderly patients: Is there cause for concern? *Journal of the American Geriatrics Society, 40,* 902–905.

Crewe, H. K., Lennard, M. S., Tucker, G. T., Woods, F. R., & Haddock, R. E. (1992). The effect of selective serotonin reuptake inhibitors on cytochrome P450 2D6 (CYP2D6) activity in human liver microsomes. *British Journal of Clinical Pharmacology, 34,* 262–265.

Druckenbrod, R., & Mulsant, B. H. (1994). Fluoxetine-induced syndrome of inappropriate antidiuretic hormone secretion: A geriatric case report and a review of the literature. *Journal of Geriatric Psychiatry and Neurology, 7,* 255–258.

Ereshefsky, L., Overman, G. G., & Karp, J. (1995). Current Psychotropic Dosing and Monitoring Guidelines. *Primary Psychiatry, 5,* 42–53.

Hyttel, J. (1994). Pharmacological characterization of selective serotonin inhibitors. *International Clinical Psychopharmacology, 9*(Suppl 1), 19–26.

Lawlor, B. A. (1990). Serotonin and Alzheimer's disease. *Psychiatric Annals, 20,* 567–570.

Pollock, B. G. (1994). Recent developments in drug metabolism of relevance to psychiatrists. *Harvard Review of Psychiatry, 2,* 204–213.

Pollock, B. G., Perel, J. M., Paradis, C. F., Fasicka, A. L., & Reynolds, C. F. (1994). Metabolic and physiologic consequences of nortriptyline treatment in the elderly. *Psychopharmacology Bulletin, 30,* 145–150.

Richelson, E. (1994). The pharmacology of antidepressants at the synapse: Focus on newer compounds. *Journal of Clinical Psychiatry, 55*(Suppl A), 34–39.

PART III
Toward a More Informed Public Policy

9

Death, Dying, and Assisted Suicide

RAMA P. COOMARASWAMY

The current literature, both medical and lay, is suffused with opinions about death, dying, and assisted suicide—much of it written by individuals with little or no clinical experience. The thoughts and opinions of an individual who has practiced general, thoracic, and cardiovascular surgery for over 30 years may be of interest in this escalating debate.

Many writers are subject to the impression that terminal cancer is always and inevitably a painful affliction. Pictures of agonizing and uncontrollable pain are used to justify assisted suicide. In the practice of surgery for over 30 years, I have never had a terminal patient whose pain could not be relieved by means of medication. I am sure that such exist, but they must be rare. Lest some suggest that my experience is limited, allow me to state that I was in medical practice before the fragmentation of specialties shunted terminal care into the hands of oncologists, that my experience ranged over the entire field of cancer surgery, and that even after it was common practice to refer surgically incurable patients to other specialties, many of my patients returned to me for terminal care. Let it also be clear that I am not stating that terminal patients do

Editor's note: This chapter originally appeared in the *Connecticut Medicine, 58,* pp. 551–556. Copyright © 1994 by Connecticut Medicine. Reprinted with permission of the publisher.

not suffer. All I am stating is that in most, if not all cases, the suffering due to pain can be adequately and completely eliminated. So much has this been the case that I have been able to promise my terminal patients that when living was no longer worth the effort, I would put them in the hospital and, once they had seen their "spiritual-care provider" (shades of "health-care providers"), I would not prolong the dying process (often incorrectly called "prolonging life") and would keep them pain free. It has been a promise which, to the best of my knowledge, I have never failed to fulfill.

Lest this statement be surprising, allow me to quote Dr. Saunders' work, which has been referred to in *The New Harvard Guide to Psychiatry* (Nicholi):

> When Saunders documented the exact incidence of practical problems in terminal cancer at St. Joseph's Hospital in London, she found that the three most common complaints were nausea and vomiting, shortness of breath, and dysphagia. It was striking that pain did not appear high on the problem list: With proper medication about 90% of her patients remained pain free.

There is considerable and possibly deliberate confusion in the literature between what is called "active" and "passive" euthanasia. Active euthanasia means actively killing a patient. Passive euthanasia means allowing a patient to die. There is a world of difference between the two. Actively and with full intention to kill another individual, even though it is done by the Kevorkian method, is murder. Physicians, except perhaps in Nazi Germany, have throughout history rejected such a role. Passive euthanasia is a misnomer—it is not euthanasia at all, but rather a matter of allowing nature to take its course without interference. As an older generation of physicians used to say, "Pneumonia is the old man's friend." Giving a patient large doses of pain medications may shorten his or her life—as, for example, when mild respiratory depression leads to a pulmonary infection that one elects (with the patient's and family's concurrence) not to treat. It is the principle of primary intent and secondary effect that makes the difference. In order to clarify this distinction, consider the patient who is given clozapine (assuming proper indications and so-called "informed consent") and who develops agranulocytosis that proves fatal. The legal system apart, the physician involved would never be accused of killing the patient. Or as another example, a surgeon performs an appendectomy on a pregnant patient who subsequently aborts; the surgeon is not guilty of performing an abortion.

Allow me to paint a clinical picture which is fairly typical in practice. In passing, let me also point out that an individual such as Dr. Kevorkian, who is a pathologist and not a clinician, would almost certainly not be familiar with such examples.

> The terminal patient has been admitted to the hospital floor for the last time. She is placed in "the single-bed room" at the end of the hall reserved for those with severe infections, high levels of radioactivity, or terminal disease. DNR (do not resuscitate) is placed over the door. Daily rounds are made. Younger patients with curable or interesting diseases are visited and examined, but when the house staff comes to this patient's room, if they stop at all, it is to wave briefly and rush away. As a case, such an individual is no longer of interest—she is one of medicine's failures. No effort is made to see if the patient is comfortable. The movement of bowels, dehydration, and bedsores are not checked. In similar manner, the nurses, aides, and medical students all avoid either examining or talking to the patient. The family rarely visits and then only for a few minutes—they have been through the long course of illness and are weary. The patient has for all intents and purposes been abandoned by physician, staff, and acquaintances.
>
> Orders are written by the medical student whose familiarity with pain medications is necessarily limited and who has been brought up on an educational diet that stresses the addictive quality of narcotics. God forbid that the terminal patient should have addiction added to her woes. Despite the fact that it is well known that terminal patients can self-administer their pain medications—usually at lower doses—better than medical personnel, rarely are they given the opportunity to do so. I cannot begin to count the number of times I have insisted that the nurse give a patient pain medication *now,* and not when she makes medication rounds.
>
> But the opposite can also happen. As evening wears on and darkness closes in, our frightened and abandoned patient begins to groan. Cries of "doctor" and "nurse" become annoying and keep the healthier patients awake. An immediate assumption is made that the cause is pain. PRN (on demand) pain medications have been ordered and the nurse comes in to give her a shot. Rarely does the nurse ask what the patient really wants. How often it is something as simple as changing the sheets because the bedpan was not brought when requested—and the patient was too weak and exhausted to maintain bladder control. The shot takes effect and 30

minutes later the patient is asleep. Quiet once again reigns on the floor. And so the patient is caught on the horns of a dilemma. Pain relief is frequently inadequate or narcotics are inappropriately administered.

There are those who will claim I have painted a highly exaggerated picture of callousness and insensitivity. Unfortunately, it has been my experience that such is all too often the case. (My own experience ranges from inner-city hospitals in the Bronx to some of the finest hospitals in Fairfield County.) There are, of course, exceptions and many mitigating circumstances that vary from hospital to hospital. For example, nurses now are so committed to paperwork that they rarely have time for what is called "primary nursing care." The net effect is that when a patient rings the bell, it is usually a nurse's aide who responds—an individual with inadequate training for the task. Yet the fact remains that whenever feasible, I ordered private nurses whom I personally knew for my postoperative and terminal patients—often telling the family that it was the greatest gift they could give a loved one.

Even though a patient can be kept pain free, this by no means guarantees she will not suffer. But what in fact is the nature of this suffering? One can categorize suffering as being on three levels—physical, psychological, and spiritual. First of all there is physical suffering resulting from the failure to be sure that such a mundane thing as adequate pain medication is given. Then there is the suffering secondary to the disease or treatment process. What is often forgotten is that pain medications are constipating and patients who are in a weakened condition because of their illness need help in moving their bowels. Terminal patients frequently get dehydrated and have long since exhausted their venous access for intravenous fluids. Interventions such as keeping the patient adequately hydrated by means of a subclavian line or Hickman catheter are frequently seen as surgical procedures and therefore rejected. Yet patients are eternally grateful for such lines, not only because they prevent the discomfort of dehydration, but also because they allow for the drawing of blood samples (often not really necessary, but God forbid the patient should die out of electrolyte balance) without being repeatedly stuck. The placement of such lines does not require that they be used for nutritional purposes. Again, few things are more disconcerting to a patient and family than the inability to clear secretions that cause the death rattle. However, gentle intermittent suctioning can easily relieve this. Mouth care is often ignored. Terminal patients rarely have the energy to brush their teeth. Continuous breathing through the mouth leads to the caking of secretions over the entire mucosal surface. Wiping out a person's mouth with a damp face cloth (not just wiping their lips with lemon sticks) can be source of great comfort. There are obviously hundreds of things that can be done to make a person's "passing" more comfortable. One hopes that when one's own time comes they will not be forgotten.

Psychological suffering is harder to define because it borders on the spiritual. However, within this category I would include depression. Many terminal patients—regardless of whether their course is short or long— become depressed. Our society's vaunted values—"He who has the most toys when he dies wins"—obviously excludes the majority from departing with a sense of accomplishment. Broken families have become the norm and tragic scenes are often played out at the deathbed. That terminal illness can be a time for reconciliation is often forgotten, and relatives have to be instructed in the need to forgive and to let go. Active and successful individuals often feel their usefulness is over and begin to see themselves as a burden on survivors. It is important to realize that medications given to the elderly can actually be the cause of depression; for example, antihypertensives given to the elderly frequently cause impotence which is experienced as "castrating." And finally, there is frank clinical depression which frequently goes untreated because it is seen as part of the disease process. A recent article in the *Connecticut Medicine* describes this situation in a patient with Alzheimer's disease very well. Individuals who see their independence and ability to function slipping away understandably are subject to depression and can be greatly helped with appropriate medications.

Third to be considered is spiritual suffering. It has been adequately demonstrated in both the psychiatric and religious literature that people do not change their personalities on the approach of death—selfish individuals remain selfish to the very end. Yet faced with death, there are few if any who do not have a sense of dread. Perhaps, after all, the religious teachings of our childhood are correct? Perhaps there will be a judgment of some sort—or even worse—perhaps there is nothing but an abysmal void. People used to die at home surrounded by praying family and friends and provided with the consolations of religion. Now they die in sterile hospitals, narcotized and frequently alone in the middle of the night with the television set or Muzac blaring. Clergy, who once spent time with the patient, now see their role as one of giving psychological support to the survivors. (Funerals have frequently become "happy times" that deprive survivors of the psychological need to mourn and to bury the past.) Yet clinicians often observe that it is the truly religious whose passing is the easiest on themselves and others. The most difficult situations I have encountered are those in which the patient and family adamantly believe in nothing.

But spiritual preparation for a patient's passing starts long before she enters the final phase. It is here that a physician can play a major role— not only if that physician himself has come to terms with his own mortality. In the absence of clergy willing to undertake this task, the physician's role becomes even more important. This brings us back to the first time when one must face the patient with bad news. One doesn't start by telling the patient everything, but rather what he or she can absorb. Three things are essential: (1) One never lies to the patient, for how can a dying patient trust a physician who lies? Families may ask the physician not to tell the patient, but can usually be convinced that such a stance is cruel. It isolates the patient who intrinsically knows something is wrong and can "smell" the insincerity of those who deny it. I have never known a patient who is dying not to have some awareness of the fact. It further prevents the person from resolving conflicts, paying debts, and putting her affairs in order. Muslim patients are particularly sensitive about dying in debt. Finally, it prevents the individual from preparing to die and virtually cuts her off from any available spiritual help. How, after all, can a patient talk to her pastor about death when assured that death is not in the offing? Many people desire a sudden and unexpected death. It may surprise those brought up in the West that other cultures consider sudden death a tragedy. Death is seen as one of the most important events in a person's life, and proper preparation for it is considered essential. Telling the patient the truth is important even on the practical level. I well remember a patient who was not informed that he had lymphoma because the physician felt it was a highly curable disease. The patient did well for several months and then cashed in his life insurance in order to expand his business. He then developed a recurrence which was unresponsive to therapy. The net result was that his business fell apart, and when he died, his wife was left financially destitute. (2) One always leaves the patient with hope. The hope for remission or cure is never false. Clinicians well know the impossibility of predicting when an individual will reach the end of his course—every bellshaped curve has two tails. Medical advances are always in the offing, and even apart from what science may have to offer, we have all seen those cases of spontaneous remission that cannot be explained. Part of this hope may be tied to prayer and pilgrimage. The physician must remember that his own agnosticism is not to be fostered on the patient. Hence it is that I have often encouraged patients who raise the issue to visit places like Lourdes or Loretto. Hindus, Jews, and Moslems also have locations where they may seek a cure. Whatever one believes about the medical effects of such actions, their psychological benefits can be immense. (3) I have always assured the patients that I would be there for them. Even when it becomes necessary to pass the patient's care on to another specialty, I have stressed my availability—especially when they have the need to talk. Finally, as the disease progresses, always depending upon what the patient is ready to hear, I have shared with them increasing details about what they are going through and what they can expect. Some patients wish to investigate alternative methods of treatment. I have investigated these with them and encouraged them to try those which we have together concluded are not likely to be harmful. For example, I well remember a patient with terminal cancer of the lung that had invaded the trachea, who wished to get vitamin therapy in Bermuda. His general condition was quite good except when the tumor encroached on his ability to breathe. As he was living out his time during a dreary winter in New York City, I encouraged him to go. He would return every four to six weeks for laser treatment of his tracheal tumor. He was, incidentally, an avid golfer.

Suffering is by no means always a curse—indeed it can be a blessing. It recalls to us our frailty and when pointing to termination, allows us to reorient our lives and place first things first. Interpersonal relationships have often been sacrificed in the pursuit of economic success and the warning which suffering offers allows for fences to be mended. There is often a fairly long period after the diagnosis is made during which the patient is asymptomatic. I usually try to find out what the patient's lifelong "dream" has been—a trip to the place of his birth—a cruise with his spouse to Alaska. It is during this period that I encourage them to fulfill such dreams. Those who take advantage of these opportunities have a chance to reflect on their lives and round patients off with a certain sense of fulfillment. It is far easier to let go at the end if one's dreams have been fulfilled.

Beware the family that wants "everything done" for the dying relative. They are often those who have failed to keep in contact during the illness and show up for the terminal event suffused with guilt. Fortunately, one can usually talk them into a proper and supportive attitude—but clearly one cannot win every battle. Even more difficult is the patient who wants everything done. Usually such an individual is convinced that any life, no matter how difficult, is better than none. Once again, one must respect the patient's wishes. And again, one is not always free to use one's best judgment. In my experience, this rarely happens with patients one has walked through the course, but rather those that one sees for the first time because their own physician has given up. They are looking for the miracle no physician can provide.

Terminal disease can be a wonderful opportunity for the patient. The way in which he faces death can be an example to the family that is remembered with fondness. I remember a good friend, a physician, who wished to commit suicide because he felt his life was a burden on others. I was able to persuade him of the need to "play the man" for the sake of his estranged son. During the last three weeks of his life, he and his son became reconciled. To this day, the son respects and admires the courage with which his father faced the end. Suicide would have left his son with a very different memory. We must remember that suffering is part of the human condition. It is not the suffering, but what we do with it that is important.

The story of the Buddha is not without pertinence. His father had been warned that once the young prince became aware of death, disease, grief, and old age, he would renounce the world and become a monk. The father did everything possible to keep knowledge of these four things from his son, but all his efforts proved impossible. And indeed, once he became aware of them, he did renounce the kingdom and enter a spiritual path. Now, a small amount of reflection makes it clear that despite utopian imperatives, mankind can never create a society in which death, disease, grief, and old age are eliminated. Indeed, such a society, supposing it were possible, might well prove to be a horror, for it is precisely the manner in which we deal with these issues that makes us human.

It is clear that we shall all grow old and frail. Physicians have a particularly difficult time with facing ineptitude because they are so invested in doing for others. I am reminded here of a personal experience. Some years ago I broke an ankle and was restricted to bed for several days. My children, who had had a reasonably comfortable existence for many years, suddenly became my nurses, cleaning bedpans and urinals. I was intensely embarrassed by this and thought to hire a nurse. Fortunately, I realized that this would be a mistake. My fracture was a wonderful opportunity for my children to show their love—something they did with grace and thankfulness. And so it is that illness provides others with a chance to do for us. To deprive others of the opportunity for showing love is both cruel and tragic. We all have ambivalence toward others—even those closest to us. To deprive others of the opportunity of giving is to force them to hold on to these ambivalent feelings when resolution is no longer possible. The fact that I was able to visit weekly with my mother when she was dying helped her greatly. In retrospect, it helped me even more.

More on terminal care. What guidelines can we use in order to know where to draw the many lines we are forced to draw? I believe these can be summed up in four simple statements—unfortunately, their application is more difficult. But first the statements:

1. Treat every patient as if she were a member of your immediate family. Do for her what you would want done for your own.

2. Be sure your patient has had the opportunity of seeing his spiritual care provider, and then make sure that terminal care is comfortable and pain free.

3. The physician must develop the skill of determining the patient's and family's wishes about terminal care without placing the burden of guilt on them for decisions made. The physician must take upon his or her shoulders the "guilt" for deciding to "let the patient go."

4. Remember that you are not obliged to use extraordinary means to keep a patient alive.

The problem of course lies in what one means by *extraordinary means*. The use of a ventilator in a patient with Guillain-Barré syndrome would not be extraordinary means. The use of the same ventilator in a terminal lung cancer patient would be. Nutritionally feeding a person who is temporarily unable to eat is not extraordinary means, but tube feeding a brain-dead patient is. No matter how many strictures courts, administrators, or well-meaning individuals may place on us, in the last analysis it is the physician who must make the call. It is a call shared with patient (when possible), the family, and often also with their minister. Unfortunately, it often happens that *extraordinary means* are instituted before one has a full knowledge of the patient's condition. I remember a case from 30 years ago when I was a chief resident in thoracic surgery. On the medical service, a young woman with widespread metastatic inflammatory cancer of the breast which had failed to respond to every form of therapy had a sudden cardiac arrest as I was walking by. I promptly opened her chest and removed a large pulmonary embolus from her left pulmonary artery—the once well-known Trandelenberg procedure. Needless to say, I was rather proud of this achievement. The medical service insisted that the patient be transferred to my service. She lived for another three months and cursed me every day for having pulled her through. I like to think she forgave me before she died.

Patients placed on the ventilator inappropriately; that is, when in fact they are brain dead or have clearly terminal disease, can be dealt with kindly. There is no need to "pull the plug." One can simply turn the intermittent mandatory ventilation (IMV) down to four. If the patient has spontaneous respiratory activity, he will demonstrate this by continuing to breathe. If, however, the respiratory center is knocked out, an IMV of four will allow the CO_2 to build up slowly to toxic levels. How much kinder this is to the patient and family than pulling out the endotracheal tube as was done to an elderly friend of mine recently—and this in front of the man's family.

Another gentle way to go. Patients with cancer of the lung frequently develop brain metastases. This usually heralds a nine-month course. Treated with limited radio-therapy and steroids, one can return them to normal activity. Again, within the framework of all that has been said above, one can promise them an easy passing. When once again they develop neurological signs, usually the return of those they presented with initially, and assuming that other causes have been ruled out, one can simply cut the steroids. One hesitates to mention such simple things in writing, but unfortunately physicians (and house staff who usually take care of these patients) currently seem unaware of such possibilities. I do not say such things should be used for every patient—but for some and perhaps most, it is a blessing.

One must be wary of yet another pitfall. Relatives who advocate euthanasia for a loved one may be far more concerned with their own suffering than that of the patient. None of us enjoys seeing another person's suffering because, among other reasons, it reminds us of our own mortality. Perhaps this is one of the reasons that we are prone to put animals "out of their misery." But a human being is more than just a higher animal. If one believes mankind is simply the product of evolutionary forces, one destroys the entire basis for the practice of medicine. Curing the ill and succoring the weak is a direct assault on whatever evolutionary process we believe may have created us. Moreover, many cultures—specifically the Hindu and Buddhist—do not put animals out of their misery but let them die by natural processes. Animals too must be allowed to "live out their karma."

What then of suicide? There will always be those who desire such an option. But why should they involve a physician in their act? Most people—even paraplegics—are perfectly capable of committing suicide without assistance. And those few who do need help can be dispatched by trained technicians with a high-school or equivalent level of education. In a novel written about the turn of the century, Robert Hugh Benson described euthanasia centers which provided for such committees, the fulfilling of the individual's last wishes, and an appropriate setting (with music of choice) where she could die with dignity. What then is the role of the psychiatrist? In my opinion, it is clearly not to sanction the act. A psychiatrist can determine whether the patient is depressed and whether or not the individual is capable of giving informed consent—both processes with which he is familiar. (One wonders whether he will write "no psychiatric contraindication to assisted suicide"?) Further, the psychiatrist can attempt to determine whether appropriate terminal care has been provided. More, of course, can be done, for he can help the individual walk the last few miles of life. Unfortunately, most psychiatrists react to terminal disease in the same manner as their surgical and medical confreres—few are qualified to work with a patient and help him face the reality of death.

Of course, some sort of committee will have to be formed to give approval for such assisted suicides. What is surprising is that politicians and advocates for euthanasia are insisting that physicians be on these committees. I think this is inappropriate. Physicians trained to preserve life and "do no harm" are not psychologically capable of having the necessary and appropriate attitudes to allow them to advocate just the opposite. That they should be asked to make such weighty decisions, when administrators and insurance companies are actively limiting their ability to make less weighty decisions on behalf of their patients, is curious. But seriously speaking, why should such committees not be made up of lawyers, politicians, euthanasia advocates, and so-called medical ethicists? Such individuals are practical men of the world and not encumbered by the psychological effects caused by years of helping to heal others.

This last paragraph may sound slightly sarcastic. However, once again let me provide a clinical vignette. I admitted a new patient one evening who had preterminal cancer of the breast. Her rather large family wished me to perform euthanasia. My evaluation of the patient was that with proper care she could have many months of good living—and indeed this was provided. She made no personal request for euthanasia. The family, however, became so insistent as to be burdensome. As it was late and I did not wish to spend the rest of the evening dealing with this issue, I drew up a syringe of morphine and asked one of them to do the injection. They all refused and insisted it was my responsibility. When I asked them why mine rather than theirs, they could give me no answer. What is involved here then is responsibility. Why should the public, or even a patient, place the responsibility for euthanasia on the physician? There may be some physicians who want to do this, and I for one do not wish to meddle with anyone's conscience. However, physicians who wish to be involved in such actions do so as individuals and not, I hope, as physicians committed to the Hippocratic Oath. Destroying life should never be equated with the relief of suffering. The possible need for assisted suicide is in many, if not most cases, a failure on the part of health- and spiritual-care providers to relieve suffering.*

---

* Physician involvement in mercy killing is intrinsically dangerous. If the indication is the "relief of suffering," indications for mercy killing can easily be expanded to include the mentally retarded, the aged, and the incompetent—to say nothing of those we don't want around for any number of reasons.

10

The Emerging Agenda for Prevention through Research and Public Policy

GARY J. KENNEDY

To recap the critical issues from earlier chapters, neither the social nor the medical perspectives on late-life suicide are sufficient to explain the magnitude of the problem or to offer easy solutions. And the number of late-life suicides will become substantially larger even if the rates plateau. Prevalence data and the most frequently cited inferences regarding causality are equally problematic. Despite the limitations of existing research and interventions, a reasoned agenda for the prevention of late-life suicide is entirely feasible. What follows is an assessment of present scientific methods as well as proposals for new approaches. The long-term and more expensive agenda for prevention through changes in public policy closes the chapter.

RESEARCH

Case Finding Studies
These studies are crucial to demonstrate what interventions are feasible prior to testing their effectiveness. Community-oriented case finding

and referral programs, modeled on the Spokane Gatekeepers would link vulnerable individuals to evaluation and treatment. Model programs of this sort would focus on primary prevention and allow researchers to identify aspects of the intervention that seemed responsible for desirable outcomes. A reduction in presumed risk factors would be the immediate goal. These include suicidal ideation, social isolation, and untreated illness—most notably hypothyroidism, congestive heart failure, agoraphobia, depression, alcohol or sedative abuse. Reduction in suicide attempts and completions would be more difficult to demonstrate.

Case finding programs could also explore novel approaches such as outreach from religious institutions, the use of peer-aged community volunteers, entitlement workers, law enforcement. Would a friendly visitor to shepherd the identified patient through the health and social services maze be as effective as in-home care provided by psychiatric social workers and nurse clinicians? To what extent are the expertise and expense of physicians necessary to make the services effective? What constitutes quality of care in community outreach? These and other logistical questions are the subjects of qualitative as well as quantitative study.

Demonstration programs are also needed for disadvantaged and immigrant minority groups. The design for an ethnically diverse but densely populated urban center would be quite different from that designed for the widely dispersed, and even more isolated but homogeneous rural seniors. Costs of transportation in some instances are likely to exceed those allocated for personnel. As always, the stigma of mental illness, both personal and social, must be kept uppermost when considering the structure of interventions.

Model programs also offer the opportunity to refine legal and ethical issues outside traditionally defined clinical contexts. When one enters the emergency room or clinic as a patient, there is an implicit contract for care evoked simply by presence in the setting. The implied consent must be made explicit when physical examination or invasive procedures are necessary. When someone else identifies the person as a patient, however, individual rights and social responsibilities are on a wholly different footing. The adult's right to privacy, the right to refuse treatment, and our public responsibility not to abandon or neglect the mentally impaired can become competing ethical imperatives. When nothing is implicit, everything is potentially coercive. Ultimately, the individual's liberty interests and the state's sovereignty interests are interdependent, neither existing in isolation of the other. Case finding programs can help develop the appropriate balance between the person's right to refuse with the state's responsibility to provide. Procedural safeguards that recognize the dilemma and make the decision-making process balanced and rational should be tested in the field.

It is easy to lose sight of the strengths for the weaknesses of case finding and intervention programs. These initiatives would almost exclusively be descriptive, exploratory, local, and small scale. As such, they could be expected to demonstrate a reduction in risk factors but not a reduction in suicidal behaviors. In most cases, they would test feasibility rather than effectiveness. And without doubt, they would serve many who are not the primary focus of the studies. Nonetheless, modest expenditures would yield valuable information on ethical and legal procedures as well as costs and logistics.

Psychological Autopsy and Record Linkage Studies

These retrospective methods provide information about suicide completers. Both rely on death certificates and the auspices of medical examiners to identify cases. The psychological autopsy entails an interview of family, friends, or neighbors, and the physicians of suicide victims (Shneidman & Faberow, 1961). Record linkage studies cross-reference suicides identified by medical examiners with individuals listed in psychiatric case registers. Data on the deceased including symptoms, diagnoses, comorbidities, social support, and treatment as they relate to suicide in retrospect are made available for study (Conwell & Caine, 1991).

Unfortunately, the means of identifying cases as well as the retrospective method bias the psychological autopsy and record linkage studies toward finding depression as the major factor contributing to completed suicide in late life. Suicidal deaths among physically ill individuals, whether the illness is acute, chronic, terminal, or self-limiting are less likely to be reported as suicidal given the stigma and the uncertainty about the contribution of the illness. A lethal ingestion of prescribed medications may require relatively few pills for seriously ill persons but amount to suicide nonetheless. Also, collateral informants may be more likely to report illness, alcohol, and depression than other social factors that might implicate themselves in the web of causality. In cases where the methods of death were less lethal than firearms, hanging, jumping from heights, or self-poisoning, the identification of a suicide by the medical examiner is less likely. As a consequence, studies of coroner's cases are less informative about the more frequent suicide attempts that do not lead to fatality, and about the phenomena of suicidal thoughts and feelings not traditionally associated with depressive disorders.

Although psychological autopsies and record linkage studies indicate that depressive disorders are the overwhelming category of mental illness associated with completed suicide in late life, questions regarding the contribution of anxiety and quasi-psychotic symptoms remain. Also in question is the extent to which suicidal presentations of mental illness are in some way atypical, more difficult to identify. Because so many suicides have seen their physician within 24 hours to 1 month before death, the psychological autopsy should be directed at determining what physician or patient behaviors prevented the realization of imminent suicide. Psychological autopsy and record linkage methods could develop a more effective risk profile for use by primary care physicians.

Case/Cohort Studies

Such studies compare psychiatric patient cases of suicide or suicidal thoughts or behavior with a cohort of nonsuicidal persons, most often other psychiatric patients. The method covers a larger group than psychological autopsy or record linkage studies by including both those who have thought about or attempted suicide and, in prospective designs, those who complete suicide. Both cross-sectional and longitudinal comparisons are possible. Particularly with hospitalized cases, the exploration of personality, neuropsychological, and biological contributions to suicidality can be explored with relative convenience. Issues of state versus trait characteristics can be studied as the patient recovers from the acute episode of illness. This method seems ideal to study individuals with manifest risk for subsequent suicide (those with prior attempts).

Case/Cohort studies might also be employed to identify secondary and tertiary preventive measures for patients receiving psychiatric services following a suicide attempt or expression of suicidal thoughts. Rehabilitative strategies for both the restoration and maintenance of physical function should be explored as a means of lessening older psychiatric patients' sense of helplessness in the face of debilitating physical illness. Psychoeducational approaches and family therapy might be explored to assist the family in returning to a more satisfying equilibrium in the aftermath of treatment for their relative's suicidality. Similarly the prevention of recurrence or the containment of incomplete response to antidepressant therapies could be explored as well as the long-term efficacy of cognitive, interpersonal, and group psychotherapy in minimizing the patient's predisposition to suicidal thought.

Studies of identified patients also provide an opportunity to refine legal and ethical precepts. The exploration of ethical dilemmas in the clinical context would better prepare us for the less clear-cut situation of case finding services in community settings. Because suicide is so frequently linked to depressive disorder in late life, a comparison of late-life depressives with and without a history of suicidal attempts and ideas would also be desirable. Biological factors and other characteristics discriminating one group from another might best be approached among a clinical sample of older depressives. With the emergence of imaging techniques that display the dynamics of neurotransmitter function as well as brain structure, the contribution of the dopaminergic system to suicidality might be explored. The serotonergic system is more often implicated in suicide, but given the distorted perceptions of physical illness identified among older suicides of the psychological autopsy studies, investigation of the dopaminergic system seems warranted.

In summary, the case/cohort approach capitalizes on the obvious risk population, allows for in-depth assessment because it has a more captive audience, can identify the therapeutic components that might minimize subsequent risk and suggest further pharmacological avenues for intervention (e.g., the indications for attacking the dopaminergic system). The weaknesses of the case/cohort method are several. Like the psychological autopsy method, it focuses on identified psychiatric patients, who represent a minority of older adults at risk. It offers little information about the unselected population of older community residents who keep their suicidal ideas secret. And it may not improve the approach to patients who have voiced suicidal ideas to their primary care providers but do not come to the attention of mental health specialists.

Longitudinal Epidemiological Study

A study of completed or attempted suicide among a nationally representative sample of the elderly would be premature given the difficulties of defining suicidal behaviors, the rarity of suicidal events, and the expense. A more fruitful approach to the epidemiology of late-life suicide may be to study suicidal ideas, at present the only reliable risk factor beyond previous attempt that could be used to segregate a population for comparison and ultimately for prevention. The applications of such a survey are several. First is the identification of risk factors for primary intervention as well as countervailing forces that are associated with freedom from risk. Second, a longitudinal epidemiological survey would provide an estimate of the prevalence, persistence, and health significance of suicidal thought. And the method need not be applied to a nationally representative sample to be informative. A single-site epidemiological survey would pilot methods that could be expanded to a more widely representative population. It would use a reasonable proxy measure of suicide, suicidal thought rather than behavior, and would be modest in costs compared with the massive Epidemiologic Catchment Area program and Established Populations for the Epidemiologic Study of the Elderly.

The weaknesses of the epidemiological study are first that it ignores feasibility and effectiveness of interventions. Second, there is no guarantee that results would satisfactorily apply to other communities. Oversampling of minorities would be required. And to yield the greatest likelihood of results at the lowest cost, it would be necessary to identify a high-risk, densely populated urban community in which advanced age and social isolation were relatively frequent. Nonetheless, the techniques to ensure adequate response rates and to reduce biases due to sampling procedures are available as are analytic methods suited to large longitudinal databases with varied predictors and outcomes of interest. Inferences regarding social isolation, physical illness and disability, psychopathology, and health care utilization could be tested prospectively. The critical questions are (a) what are the correlates and predictors of suicidal thought, (b) what is the associated morbidity and mortality?

EDUCATION AS THE PUBLIC POLICY PRIORITY

The immediate public policy priorities in prevention are first educational and second legislative. If physicians, clergy, and seniors themselves are the sentinels, how well are our institutions educating them and how well is the media informing them? A public relations campaign to better inform senior citizens about the role of depression in suicide and about the safety and effectiveness of antidepressant medications is indicated. Seniors should be enlisted in preventive programs, not just to lessen their peers' isolation but to identify potential victims of suicide. Sources of referral for individuals whom seniors identify as isolated and disabled would also be potentially useful. Lectures at senior citizen centers, churches, and synagogues may miss the most vulnerable, isolated people at risk but seem likely to demystify late-life suicide and would perhaps have a halo effect in the community of older adults. Educational offerings by and for the clergy should also be carried out.

Physicians need education to lower their threshold for treating depression. Early and ongoing treatment of mental illness is primary, secondary, and tertiary prevention of late-life suicide. Regarding treatment, there is a wide choice of safe and effective treatments for depression and anxiety. However, most individuals who might benefit are not identified or offered treatment, or are not sufficiently treated. Depression tends to be a persistent illness characterized by periods of recovery and recurrence. Comorbidity of mental and physical illness is the rule rather than the exception in late life. When physical complaints of illness do not conform to the usual patterns of geriatric syndromes and disorders, a collateral informant may be the most effective means of identifying signs and symptoms of mental illness.

Educating the press about late-life suicide is a relatively straightforward step toward reducing the suicide rate. Examples of the responsible portrayal of older adult suicide are available. A greater emphasis on treatable depression rather than immutable social forces as influencing suicide would be desirable. Efforts to demystify suicide, which are common in teenage suicide prevention programs, should be extended to reports of late-life suicide. Efforts to reduce late-life suicides will have an impact on the suicidal risk of future generations by preventing suicide from becoming a bitter family legacy.

The combined costs of educational programs for the public, press, physicians, and clergy would be prohibitive. However, a number of foundations whose interests have historically focused on suicide or senior citizens might mount the effort provided the rationale is clear. Spokespersons from these groups should respond to those who are championing suicide and euthanasia to counter the suggestion that late-life suicide is an acceptable solution to fears of helplessness.

LEGISLATION AND HEALTH
CARE REFORMS

At the same time, physicians and legislators must develop better laws as well as clinical practices to ensure the older person's autonomy. The Patient Self-Determination Act (Omnibus Budget Reconciliation Act of 1990) should be a more prominent standard of clinical practice, as routine as the annual assessment. The time needed to discuss these sensitive, difficult decisions (Wolf et al., 1991) should be reimbursed as a separate Medicare procedure.

Reduction in the availability of lethal means (handgun control) should also be attempted through legislation as well as educating physicians that firearms in the household represent a substantial risk for suicide among older adults. Reducing the lethality of suicidal methods may not decrease the morbidity but should reduce the mortality of suicide attempts. Even if other methods are substituted so that the attempt rate does not fall, the net effect would still be beneficial.

Concerns over the growing costs of health entitlements and universal access to care threaten to displace the need for changes in public policy that might reduce late-life suicide. However, the crisis in health care need not override the relatively modest cost of research. Data rather than assertions are needed on present clinical practice and public preferences, as well as epidemiology. Competition for existing research funds will ensure that only efficient designs get funded.

We also need better terminology for public discourse. Is the right to die in the context of intractable pain or shortness of breath the same

---

TABLE 10–1
The Emerging Agenda for Prevention Through Research and Public Policy

---

- Small scale case-finding studies to demonstrate what is logistically feasible for providers and what is acceptable to individuals and the community. The focus would be sociodemographic indicators of presumed rather than established risk.

- Case/cohort studies to identify the biological, neuropsychological, and diagnostic attributes of patient groups with suicidal ideas or behavior and to determine the efficacy and specificity of psychotherapy and pharmacotherapy. The focus would be persons at relatively high, identified risk.

- Psychological autopsy studies to explore primary-care physician's difficulties with case identification and the presentation of potentially reversible but cloaked factors among suicide completers. The focus would be individuals who in hindsight were at highest risk.

- Longitudinal epidemiological studies to identify the correlates and predictors of suicidal thought as a proxy measure for suicidal behavior and to estimate the morbidity and mortality of suicidal thought as a means of gauging its clinical significance and indications for intervention. The full spectrum of risk could be validated with measures of morbidity and mortality.

- Public policy should focus first on educating the religious and health professions and the media about the link between treatable mental illness and suicidality. Advocacy groups might offset costs of a public relations campaign that would otherwise be prohibitive and provide venues for a more informed debate about suicide and euthanasia.

- Public policy should strive to ensure that the Patient Self-Determination act is an integral component of primary care and is not overly burdened by regulation and documentation. Legislation to reduce the use of firearms for suicide should be passed.

---

as the right to suicide in less compelling circumstances? Can we avoid legitimizing suicide if we continue to ignore the duality of social and psychopathological causation in less than desperate situations? How do we escape the ethical conflict of discussing late-life euthanasia in the context of cutting the expense of late-life health care? If the accessibility and quality of care, particularly mental health care for older adults is problematic, can physician-assisted suicide be any less so? As a result of these and other questions, a statement of consensus will require time to evolve. There should be no rush to consensus given the present flux in health care funding and the lack of better clinical science. Ultimately, effective policy will incorporate social, psychopathological, legal, and ethical dimensions of the problem.

The movement toward universal health care will require clinical scientists to identify high-risk groups in whom defined interventions are reasonably effective while preserving liberty. Managed competition must not be allowed to abandon suicidal older adults who do not seek care because of apathy or fatalism associated with depressive disorders. Finally, the growing wealth of treatments and increasing sophistication of geriatric training and research promise to lessen the morbidity and mortality of suicidal behavior in late life. Older Americans should accept nothing less. Table 10–1 summarizes the agenda described in this chapter.

REFERENCES

Conwell, Y., & Caine, E. D. (1991). Suicide in the elderly chronic patient population. In E. Light & B. D. Lebowitz (Eds.), *The elderly with chronic mental illness* (pp. 31–52). New York: Springer.

Omnibus Budget Reconciliation Act of 1990, Pub. L. No. 101-508, §§4206, 4751 (codified in scattered sections of 42 U.S.C., especially §§1395cc, 1396a (West Supp. 1991)).

Shneidman, E. S., & Farberow, N. L. (1961). Sample investigations for equivocal deaths. In N. L. Farberow & E. S. Shneidman (Eds.), *Cry for help* (pp. 118–129). New York: McGraw-Hill.

Wolf, S. M., Boyle, P., Callahan, D., Fins, J. J., Jennings, B., Nelson, J. L., Barondess, J. A., Brock, D. W., Dresser, R., & Emanuel, L. (1991). Sources of concern about the Patient Self-Determination Act. *New England Journal of Medicine, 325,* 1666–1671.

Author Index

Subject Index

169

Risk assessment:
  diagnosis-precipitated suicide, 106–107
  "exclusiveness" myth, 107–108
  false positives/false negatives, 108
Risk factors:
  neurobiological, 13–14
  overview, 83–90
  suicidal methods, 9
Ritalin, 135, 137

St. Louis Epidemiologic Catchment Area
    (ECA):
  depressive disorders, 25
  longitudinal epidemiological research,
    158
  major mental disorders, 14–15, 25
Saunders, Dr., 142
Secretiveness, 105
Sedation, 123–124
Sedatives, 41
Self-acceptance, 98
Self-concept, 85
Self-injury, 9
Self-neglect, 5
Self-poisoning, 155
Self-starvation, 9
Self-worth, 13
Separation anxiety, 105, 112
Separation-individuation, 27
Seppuku, 66
Serotonergic system:
  depression and, 24, 39–40, 43–44
  inferences from, 13–14, 24, 39–40
Serotonin reuptake blockers:
  function of, 45, 123–124
  types of, 136
Sertraline, 124, 135–136
Serzone, 137
Severe depression, biological treatment of:
  electroconvulsive therapy (ECT),
    126–131
  overview, 119–121
  pharmacotherapy, 121–126
Sexual drive, 105
Shortcomings, improvement strategies,
    97–98
Sinquan, 136

Social factors, assessment, 104
Social isolation, 7, 87, 104, 154
Social support, lack of, 14
Socioeconomic status, as risk factor, 5–7
Spiritual-care provider, 142
Spiritual suffering, 145–146
Stanford Geriatric Education Center, 53
State *vs.* trait, 16
Stigma, 12–13, 155
Stomach cancer, 58
Storytelling, 110
Stroke, 85
Subintentional death, 11
Substance abuse, *see* Alcohol abuse;
    Alcoholism; Drug abuse
Substitution, 97
Succinylcholine, 130
Suffocation, 9
Suicidal ideation, 154
Suicidality:
  measurement of, 92
  neurobiology of, 13–14
Suicidal talk, 14
Suicidal thought, 12, 15, 96–97, 156
Suicide attempts, 4–5, 15, 87
Suicide methods, 8–9
Suicide pacts, 115
Suicide prevention:
  psychotherapeutic approach to, 108–109
  research and public policy agenda,
    153–161
Suicide rates, generally, 4–5
Suicide Risk Scale (SRS), 92–93
Suspicion, 16

Tardive dyskinesia, 125–127
Tausk, Victor, 113
Teenage suicide, *see* Adolescent suicide
Terminal illness:
  care guidelines, 149
  nursing care, 144–145
  pain and suffering, 141–142
  physician's role, 146–149
  psychological suffering, 145
  as risk factor, 13
  spiritual preparation, 146–147
  spiritual suffering, 147–148